ABC of
Clinical Resilience

ABC of

Clinical Resilience

EDITED BY

Anna Frain
University of Nottingham
Nottingham, UK

Sue Murphy
University of British Columbia
Vancouver, Canada

John Frain
University of Nottingham
Nottingham, UK

WILEY Blackwell

This edition first published 2021
© 2021 John Wiley & Sons Ltd

The right of Anna Frain, Sue Murphy and John Frain to be identified as the authors of the editorial material in this work has been asserted in accordance with law.

Registered Office(s)
John Wiley & Sons, Inc., 111 River Street, Hoboken, NJ 07030, USA
John Wiley & Sons Ltd, The Atrium, Southern Gate, Chichester, West Sussex, PO19 8SQ, UK

Editorial Office
9600 Garsington Road, Oxford, OX4 2DQ, UK

For details of our global editorial offices, customer services, and more information about Wiley products, visit us at www.wiley.com.

Wiley also publishes its books in a variety of electronic formats and by print-on-demand. Some content that appears in standard print versions of this book may not be available in other formats.

Library of Congress Cataloging-in-Publication Data

Names: Frain, Anna, editor. | Murphy, Sue (Physical therapist), editor. |
    Frain, John (John Patrick James), editor.
Title: ABC of clinical resilience / edited by Anna Frain, Sue Murphy, John
    Frain.
Other titles: ABC series (Malden, Mass.)
Description: First edition. | Hoboken, NJ : Wiley-Blackwell, 2021. |
    Series: ABC series | Includes bibliographical references and index.
Identifiers: LCCN 2020054591 (print) | LCCN 2020054592 (ebook) | ISBN
    9781119693437 (paperback) | ISBN 9781119693475 (adobe pdf) | ISBN
    9781119693444 (epub)
Subjects: MESH: Interprofessional Relations | Empathy | Resilience,
    Psychological | Clinical Medicine
Classification: LCC RC46 (print) | LCC RC46 (ebook) | NLM W 62 | DDC
    616–dc23
LC record available at https://lccn.loc.gov/2020054591
LC ebook record available at https://lccn.loc.gov/2020054592

Cover Design: Wiley
Cover Image: © serts/E+/Getty Images

Set in 9.25/12pt Minion by SPi Global, Pondicherry, India
Printed and bound by CPI Group (UK) Ltd, Croydon, CR0 4YY

C9781119693437_060521

Contents

Contributors

John Ballatt, FRCGP (Hon)

Director, The Openings Consultancy, Leicester, UK

Julie Carlson, MSW, RCSW

Registered Clinical Social Worker
Fraser Developmental Clinic, British Columbia, Canada

Nicola Cooper, MBChB, FAcadMEd, FRCPE, FRACP, SFHEA

Consultant Physician & Clinical Associate Professor in Medical Education
University Hospitals of Derby & Burton NHS Foundation Trust
and
Medical Education Centre, University of Nottingham, UK

Barry Evans, BMBS (Hons), MRCP (UK)

Consultant Physician
University Hospitals of Derby & Burton NHS Foundation Trust, UK

Anna Frain, MBChB, MRCGP, PGCert Medical Education

General Practitioner Partner
GP Teaching Fellow, University of Nottingham Graduate Entry Medical School
Programme Director, Derby Speciality Training Programme for General Practice, Nottingham, UK

John Frain, MB ChB, MSc, FRCGP, DCH, DGM, DRCOG, PGDipCard, AFHEA

Clinical Associate Professor & GEM Director of Clinical Skills,
Division of Medical Sciences and Graduate Entry Medicine
University of Nottingham, UK

Susanne Hewitt, MBE, MBChB (Hons), FRCS, FRCEM

Consultant Emergency Medicine
University Hospitals of Derby & Burton NHS Foundation Trust, UK

Carrie Krekoski, RDH, BDSc (Dental Hygiene), MEd

Practice Education Manager
Office of the Vice President, Health
University of British Columbia, Canada

Sue Murphy, BHSc (PT), MEd

Faculty of Medicine, Department of Physical Therapy
University of British Columbia, Vancouver Campus, Canada

Lynn Musto, PhD, RN, RPN

Assistant Professor
School of Nursing, Trinity Western University, British Columbia, Canada

Sarah Nicholls, BSc, BMBS

Junior Doctor, Emergency Department
Queens Medical Centre, Nottingham, UK

Betsabeh Parsa, BEd, MEd

Faculty of Medicine, Department of Physical Therapy
University of British Columbia, Vancouver Campus, Canada

Carla Stanton, BMBS, BMedSci, MRCGP, PgDip, DPD

General Practitioner
Functional Medicine Doctor, Hertfordshire, UK

Victoria Wood, MA

Strategic Lead, Health Systems
Office of the Vice President, Health
University of British Columbia, Canada

Preface

'To err is human' but so is to excel. Resilience recognises this. It is about bouncing back, regaining our shape – about not merely carrying on, but becoming more self-aware rather than more self-critical. Clinical resilience is not about standing apart from our patients but embracing the humanity we share and planning for the physical, emotional and cognitive effects our work has upon us. Our work is intense, and it is a paradox of modern healthcare systems that, despite the incredible treatment pathways and technological advances we have achieved, our most precious resource – those who deliver the care – report feeling increasingly burned out and unable to carry on.

We are human beings trying to help other human beings. Our professional role often requires us to be bigger than who we believe we are capable of being. When we fall short of this self-imposed expectation, many of us feel we have failed, that we have let ourselves down as well as our patients and our colleagues. Though we must be aware of our limitations, we should not be bound by them.

A recurring theme of this book is the need in healthcare for greater kindness. Not kindness as simply an emotional feeling – important though this is – but intelligent kindness, the kindness that motivates us to be cooperative rather than competitive with one another; to feel connected, thoughtful and with a sense of kinship towards other people. This connectedness starts with thoughtfulness towards ourselves, and learning about the impact on our physiology and our cognitive performance of the stressful environments in which we are all working. The potential gains are substantial. First, there is our own well-being, and a recovery of that 'joy of practice' which first alerted us to the attraction and fulfilment of working in healthcare. Secondly, greater safety and well-being of staff means improved safety for patients and a reduction in the medical error related to staff burnout. There is a particular responsibility on healthcare regulators, leaders and providers to develop the intelligent kindness towards healthcare staff which has too often been absent, so that staff and their patients remain safe.

We are grateful for the contribution of our authors, all of whom committed to this project before the outset of the Covid-19 pandemic, an event which has bought into much sharper focus so many of the themes we set out to explore in this book. They have shown resilience in completing their chapters in such a timely way despite the challenging circumstances. We work in Canada and the UK, and so this book inevitably reflects perspectives on resilience in our particular countries. However, from our professional conversations, we believe the themes we have explored reflect concerns in many countries and health systems worldwide.

We hope the individual reader will find this book of interest. With our emerging understanding of resilience and its importance to patient care, training programmes are increasingly considering how to incorporate resilience into healthcare education. We hope our work will be helpful to them as well.

Anna Frain
Sue Murphy
John Frain
February 2021

CHAPTER 1

Why resilience? Why now?

Anna Frain[1], Sue Murphy[2], and John Frain[3]

[1] University of Nottingham, Graduate Entry Medical School, Derby Speciality Training Programme for General Practice, Nottingham, UK
[2] Faculty of Medicine, Department of Physical Therapy, University of British Columbia, Vancouver Campus, Canada
[3] Division of Medical Sciences and Graduate Entry Medicine, University of Nottingham, UK

OVERVIEW

- Those entering healthcare professions are motivated by the potential 'joy of practice'.
- Healthcare practitioners are being harmed by the impact of the systems in which they work.
- *Burnout* is an occupational hazard for all healthcare workers and increases the risks of both major and minor errors in caring for patients.
- Equality and inclusion in healthcare are not only morally right but enables all to fulfil their potential to improve patient outcomes and maintain practitioner well-being.
- The Covid-19 pandemic has brought into sharper focus the impact and current challenges of the working environment upon healthcare workers.
- Organisations have a duty of care to protect patient safety by supporting healthcare workers with intelligent kindness.

Introduction

Healthcare workers are human beings trying to help other human beings. This invariably leads to a discussion of human frailty and shortcomings. Yet, the skills and abilities of practitioners are awesome, and we often have an insufficient sense of awe regarding them – to listen and to understand the effects of suffering on patients, to use our senses to examine and to diagnose, to provide comfort and support, to restore to health, to witness both the greatest joys in patients' lives as well as their darkest moments. Undoubtedly, this work requires the full use of our talents and is rewarded by the joy of practice.

Alongside this, advances in treatments across the multidisciplinary spectrum of healthcare in the past century enables us to do more and achieve more for patients and to genuinely feel we are making a difference to peoples' lives. Those entering healthcare training should be confident they are entering an occupation at the cutting edge of human endeavour and characterised by the sense of the well-being and resilience of those working in it.

Yet, the reality for many practitioners is very different. Confronted by the uncertainties and ambiguities of practice as well as the stresses of the healthcare environment, new entrants to the professions show increased reluctance to undertake specialty training, deciding to take career breaks or leave the profession completely (Figure 1.1). This established problem is so significant and widespread that it must be considered to genuinely threaten the future sustainability of modern healthcare. *Resilience* implies an ability to 'bounce back', to regain our well-being after a distorting experience. The data suggests we are not bouncing back as well as perhaps we once did. This is impacting patient care and providing immeasurable harm to healthcare providers.

'First, do no harm'

For UK healthcare professions, the past decade is bookended by two events. First, a private citizen's Freedom of Information request in 2012 led to the publication of an internal review by the General Medical Council (GMC) which revealed that, during the 2005–2013 period, 28 doctors had committed suicide whilst undergoing the GMC's fitness-to-practice (FTP) investigations (Horsfall, 2014). Casey and Choong argued that these deaths were preventable and the GMC has a duty of care towards doctors under investigation (Casey and Choong, 2016) (Box 1.1).

Practitioner suicide and distress is not unique to the UK, nor is it confined to doctors (Hofmann, 2018). Nonetheless, these healthcare professionals likely entered training with the same aspirations and hopes as their peers. In their deaths, they left behind people who loved and needed them. A healthcare culture which seemingly leaves people viewing suicide as their only alternative should concern us all – as John Dunne said, 'Any man's death diminishes me, because I am involved in Mankind'.

Second, the initial phase in the UK of the Covid-19 pandemic was characterised by shortages of personal protective equipment (PPE), with the result that staff felt they were being required either to place themselves at risk without adequate protection, or to decline to care for patients and risk disciplinary action. This

---

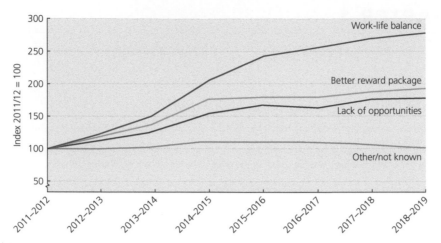

Figure 1.1 Change in reason for leaving given by staff (for voluntary resignations), 2011–2012 to 2018–2019 (Index at 2011/2012 = 100). Source: The Health Foundation (2019). © 2019, The Health Foundation.

impression of a lack of concern for healthcare staff reached its apotheosis when a prominent UK politician suggested that shortages of PPE were occurring due to wasteful usage by healthcare staff (see Chapter 6). Subsequently, reports emerged of higher-risk staff feeling unable to request the PPE *to which they were entitled*.

On a more mundane level, healthcare staff report day-to-day shortages in their work in terms of access to food, rest breaks and adequate on-call facilities, such that these provisions are not in step with employment law (GMC, 2019). Even a cursory look at Maslow's triangle (Chapter 3) suggests that meeting a practitioner's basic psychological and physical needs is required to safeguard and provide support for the high-level problem-solving necessary in clinical decision-making; it is unlikely that depriving people of food, drink and adequate rest improves patient safety. When we consider clinical resilience, it is important that we do not impose on practitioners yet another burden of fearing failure. Rather, it is about enabling clinicians to optimise their cognitive performance,

be the best they can be and recover the joy of practice. In this, organisations have a particular responsibility (Chapter 8). With resilience, our recurring theme is kindness. Kind health systems and organisations will more greatly facilitate the potential of their teams and the safety of patients.

Increasing patient expectations, complaints and litigation

Zuzsanna Jakab (WHO) emphasises that peoples' expectations of healthcare have changed, and that they wish for greater involvement in their healthcare, including in making decisions about treatment (Jakab, 2011). However, many health inequalities still exist and indicate a need for patient empowerment. Patients may not have the material, educational or political means to access health, now considered a basic human right.

Increasing patient expectations has led to an increasing number of complaints and litigation. In UK Primary Care, patients' written complaints about care increased by 4058 (4.5%) – from 90579 in 2016–2017 to 94637 (NHS Digital. Data on written complaints in the NHS, 2017–2018). In terms of impact on all parties, this is not sustainable. Where practitioners are unable to cope with understandable negative feelings of shock, burnout and anger following a complaint, there is a risk of post-traumatic stress disorder (PTSD), leading to their being described as a 'second victim' of the event (Chapter 4).

Maintaining resilience is challenging where a practitioner works in an organisation in which they feel undervalued and which appears to favour a culture of punishment rather than one of learning. Bourne found that complaints not only seriously impact doctors' psychological well-being but are also associated with defensive practice (Bourne *et al.*, 2016). This has a detrimental effect on patient care. Resolution of complaints and significant event analysis is essential for patient safety and service improvement. However, investigation procedures require transparency and timeliness to actually facilitate patient safety and practitioner resilience. A more resilient approach by practitioners to receiving complaints and their role in learning may then be possible to ensure better patient care.

Box 1.1 Suicide whilst under GMC's fitness to practise investigation: were those deaths preventable?

In their review of suicides whilst under the GMC's FTP procedures, Casey and Choong argued that the GMC has a duty of care towards its members and that these suicides were preventable. Coroners were also identified as having a duty to report these suicides as preventable to the GMC. However, Casey and Choong could not identify that these deaths had been reported in line with established legislation. They also commented: 'The high prevalence of suicide among physicians in general should not obscure the fact that suicide whilst under the GMC's FTP investigations is sufficiently unique and deserves special attention. It is thereby a matter of profound regret that it had to take a random FOI request by an independent party to eventually highlight just how serious and extensive the problem is. That FTP investigation has never, prior to that, been isolated and identified as a distinct risk factor for physician suicide meant that practically nothing has been done to avert such deaths'.

Source: Based on Casey and Choong (2016).

Why now?

In the twenty-first century, healthcare workers face multiple local and global challenges to their resilience. In our initial chapters, we explore the emotional impact of working in healthcare (Chapter 2). Healthcare has both challenges and rewards. These are considerable, and we are all familiar with the feeling of seeing a life saved, a goal achieved, perhaps soon followed by the despair of a tragic outcome or setback. Every interaction involves the care of – and communication with – a fellow human with needs and vulnerabilities. The fact that professionals sometimes struggle is predictable and understandable. Often, we begin practicing these skills required for these experiences at a time in our lives when we are still maturing and adapting to the emotional landscape of adulthood. Learning to empathise with the suffering of others can be difficult. In addition to this, the transition from the classroom to the uncertainties of clinical practice can engender feelings of being unable to cope and not being good enough. Often referred to as 'imposter syndrome', Gottlieb *et al.* found rates of 22–60% in physicians and physicians in training (see Chapter 4). Gender, low self-esteem and institutional culture are risk factors, while social support, validation of success, positive affirmation and personal and shared reflections were protective (Gottlieb *et al.*, 2020). Feeling unsupported as we make our first clinical decisions can only exacerbate further feelings of being a fraud. Imposter syndrome is associated with increased risk of burnout and suicide.

Our patients require us to be cognitively 'at the top of our game' during every encounter. Diagnostic error is unfortunately common, and faulty cognition is a contributor to this. Evidence from neuroscience increasingly supports a link between our mood and cognition. This was recognised not only in the context of mental health but increasingly in the context of clinical reasoning. We discuss this in Chapter 3.

In addressing our cognitive performance, we need to consider our 'career cycle' (see Chapter 4). Our physical and mental abilities change over a working lifetime. In addition, our knowledge base and clinical experience change over time. There are transitions during our career (promotions, learning new procedures, complaints, personal life events) when our resilience may be more challenged and our propensity to burnout increased (Puddester *et al.*, 2009). During these times, our likelihood of making a major mistake rises. Chapter 4 discusses these phases and strategies for coping with them.

Since the 1960s, heart rate variability (HRV) has been recognised as part of the stress response. For example, patients with depression have reduced HRV. Our stress response, of which HRV is part, evolved over thousands of years and for a different stress landscape. Change, including in healthcare, proceeds at an increasingly rapid pace, and we have not necessarily adapted to this. Many healthcare workers report practicing in a state of constant stress (NHS England, 2018). In turn, our cognitive performance and clinical decision-making is impaired. In Chapter 5, we outline the physiology of well-being.

John Donne's assertion of our being 'involved in mankind' suggests that a connection or kinship with others should be mutually beneficial for all – as Donne also wrote, 'No man is an island'.

There is a responsibility to be cooperative with others in return for a right to receive cooperation and support from others. This is an affirmation of life and is reflected in the quality our relationships with our patients and colleagues. I, as an individual, my patients, my colleagues, my employer and regulator are all involved in mankind and connected to one another. In healthcare, as in life, we can achieve more for our patients through cooperation. Our singular well-being is dependent on our working together and only brought into being by our 'intelligent kindness' towards one another. This is considered at length in Chapter 6.

The individual practitioner cannot be resilient alone, and so we have to consider the role of teams on patient care and staff resilience. Riskin *et al.* demonstrated the effect of rudeness in healthcare teams and of a culture of rudeness in the working environment, both on procedural tasks and, even more so, on the communication tasks which underpin good clinical decision-making and effective patient treatment (Riskin *et al.*, 2015). Kindness to patients improves their health outcomes. Kindness to each other improves patient safety. Organisational kindness results in resilient professionals in a safer environment with better patient outcomes. It is a virtuous circle. We discuss this further in Chapters 7 and 8. Chapter 9 looks at resilience in practice and how approaches such as the 'most respectful interpretation' in assessing the motivation and intentions of others can be transformative in the relationships of healthcare professionals both with each other and with our patients.

Equality, diversity and inclusion in healthcare resilience

We cannot consider practitioner resilience and its relationship to patient safety without acknowledging that our lofty proclamations of equality for all is far away from the lived experience of many of our colleagues. For example, in the UK National Health Service (NHS), there is a significantly higher percentage of black, Asian, minority ethnic (BAME) workers than in the general population (21% versus 13.8%). In London, while 43% of the NHS workforce is from BAME backgrounds, they occupy only 14% of board-level positions in local healthcare (Kings Fund, 2018).

Staff experiences include the following:

> '…*patients really can be difficult. I mean, recently I had a patient who told me that I was the wrong colour to be English*'
> (Kings Fund, 2019)

While initiatives such as the British Medical Association's Equality Matters campaign and the BMA Charter on Racism in Medicine have sought to address this, the extent of the problem was brought into sharper focus during the 2020 pandemic, when it emerged that the death rate among BAME healthcare workers was disproportionately higher than non-BAME practitioners (Box 1.2). This was a tragedy set against the backdrop of a health service which would collapse without BAME staff.

There is evidence that BAME staff struggled more to obtain adequate PPE as compared to their white counterparts (Box 1.3).

Box 1.2 **Proportion of Covid-19 related death in UK healthcare workers from BAME background.**

UK healthcare workers from BAME background have been disproportionately affected by the Covid-19 pandemic. This is manifested by increased death rates across groups of healthcare workers:

- 21% of all healthcare workers are BAME.
- 63% of healthcare workers who have died were BAME.
- 20% of nursing staff are BAME.
- 64% of nurses who died were BAME.
- 44% of medical staff are BAME.
- 95% of doctors who died were BAME.

Source: Adapted from HSJ Survey (2020).

Box 1.3 **Access to personal protective equipment (PPE) in UK healthcare workers from BAME background.**

A survey published by the Royal College of Nursing on 28 May 2020 found that BAME-category nursing staff were more likely to have difficulty accessing adequate PPE during the Covid-19 pandemic:

- 43% of BAME staff had enough eye and face protection, as compared to 66% of white British nursing staff.
- 37% of BAME nurses did not have enough fluid-repellent gowns, as compared to 19% of white British nurses.
- 53% of BAME respondents had been asked to reuse single-use PPE, as compared to 42% of white British respondents.
- 40% of BAME staff received training in what PPE to wear, as compared to 31% of white British respondents.

Source: Based on Royal College of Nursing (2020).

Box 1.4 **Story of Consultant Urologist, Mr Abdul Chowdhury.**

Abdul Mabud Chowdhury was a consultant urologist at Homerton University Hospital in East London. After training in Bangladesh and working in Zimbabwe, he moved to the United Kingdom to work in the NHS.

At an early stage of the Covid-19 pandemic, Mr Chowdhury appealed to the UK prime minister for 'appropriate PPE and remedies' to 'protect ourselves and our families'.

Five days later, he was admitted to hospital and subsequently died of Covid-19.

Dr Chaand Nagpaul, chairman of the British Medical Association (BMA), said it was 'so tragic' that the 53-year-old had died after issuing a warning about a lack of PPE.

Source: Based on BBC News (10 April 2020).

Box 1.5 **The role of the active bystander.**

Active bystanders show that certain types of behaviours are not widely accepted by others and break the silence that has previously allowed them to thrive. Active bystanding to address behaviour targeted at minority or marginalised groups such as BAME students is also very important in demonstrating support and inclusion.

The BMA Charter advocates an ABC approach:

Assess for safety: if you see someone in trouble, ask yourself if you can help safely in any way.

Be in a group: it is safer to call out behaviour or intervene in a group, and where this is not possible, report the behaviour to others who can act.

Care for the person who may need help and ask them if they are okay.

Source: BMA (2020).

Nowhere was this more tragically illustrated than in the case of Abdul Mabud Choudhry (Box 1.4).

How are intelligent kindness and resilience relevant here? An individual cannot be resilient in a system which fails them. Many forms of discrimination including those based on race, gender, sexual orientation and belief exist in healthcare. As individuals and organisations, we need to recognise discrimination and make changes to create a level playing field for all. An individual's resilience is challenged if their workplace is permeated by discrimination. We should be mindful that our colleagues experience many repeated ways of discrimination:

> *'Modern racism is far more subtle. It's indirect, it's oblique and it is far more difficult for others who are not on the receiving end of it to detect'.*
>
> – Professor Binna Kandola OBE

Our own growth as resilient practitioners includes being able to empathise and understand the lived experiences of those who work alongside us. The concept of whistleblowing as a component of patient safety is now well established. Alongside this, we need to embed within our professional values the need to be 'active bystanders' for our colleagues whose resilience and well-being is undermined by discrimination (Box 1.5)

> *'What hurts the victim the most is not the cruelty of the oppressor but the silence of the bystander'.*
>
> – Elie Wiesel, Holocaust survivor

Conclusion

The global pandemic has reminded us of the need to protect healthcare workers in order to enable them to optimally care for patients. A UK Institute for Public Policy Research report in April 2020 (Thomas and Quilter-Pinner, 2020) reported that half of health workers felt their mental health had deteriorated in the first eight weeks of the pandemic, and 20% reported that Covid-19 and the resulting difficulties had made them more likely to leave their profession. They suggested five core guarantees that need to be given to the health and care workforce.

- *Safety*: Staff shouldn't be under pressure to work without adequate protective equipment.
- *Accommodation*: For staff facing long journeys to work or with concerns about family safety, there should be alternative accommodation provided.
- *Mental health*: Workers' mental health should be ensured by extending priority access to health and care professionals.
- *Remuneration*: Staff should receive their full salary if they fall ill; and, beyond the pandemic, no health and care professional should be paid less than the real living wage.
- *Care guarantee*: Government should support professionals to remain in work by ensuring that they are able to meet unpaid care commitments – such as childcare or caring for other dependent family members.

Organisations need to embed these guarantees, as part of resilience training and support for practitioners to facilitate safe and effective delivery of patient care. Possible approaches to training are considered in Chapter 10.

Healthcare practitioners are motivated, almost without exception, by a desire to safely and effectively restore their patients to health and well-being. During the pandemic, this has been universally recognised by the public in a myriad of forms – from a weekly round of communal applause to feats of extraordinary fundraising to support local staff. They deserve the thanks and respect of us all:

> *'It is not the critic who counts; nor the man who points out how the strong man stumbles, or where the doer of deeds could have done them better. The credit belongs to the man who is actually in the arena, whose face is marred by dust and sweat and blood; who strives valiantly; who errs, who comes short again and again, because there is no effort without error and shortcoming...'*
>
> – Theodore Roosevelt

Further reading/resources

BBC News (2020) Coronavirus: NHS doctor who pleaded for PPE dies, 10 April 2020. bbc.co.uk (accessed 8.11.2020).

Bourne, T., Vanderhaegen, J., Vranken, R., *et al.* (2016) Doctors' experiences and their perception of the most stressful aspects of complaints processes in the UK: an analysis of qualitative survey data. *BMJ Open*, **6** (7), e011711. DOI: 10.1136/bmjopen-2016-011711. PMID: 27377638; PMCID: PMC4947769.

British Medical Association (BMA) (2020). *A Charter for Medical Schools to Prevent and Address Racial Harassment*. British Medical Association, UK.

Casey, D. and Choong, K. A. (2016) Suicide whilst under GMC's fitness to practise investigation: were those deaths preventable? *Journal of Forensic and Legal Medicine*, **37**, 22–27. DOI: 10.1016/j.jflm.2015.10.002. Epub 2015 Oct 22. PMID: 26519926.

General Medical Council (GMC). (2019) *Caring for Doctors; Caring for Patients*. General Medical Council, UK.

Gottlieb, M., Chung, A., Battaglioli, N., *et al.* (2020) Impostor syndrome among physicians and physicians in training: a scoping review. *Medical Education*, **54** (2), 116–124. DOI: 10.1111/medu.13956. Epub 2019 Nov 6. PMID: 31692028

The Health Foundation (2019) *Falling Short: The NHS Workforce Challenge*. The Health Foundation, UK.

Hofmann, P. B. (2018) Stress among healthcare professionals calls out for Attention. *Journal of Healthcare Management*, **63** (5), 294–297. DOI: 10.1097/JHM-D-18-00137. PMID: 30180024.

Horsfall, S. (2014) *Doctors Who Commit Suicide While Under GMC's FTP Investigation*. The General Medical Council.

HSJ Survey (2020). Adapted from COVID-19: the risk to BAME doctors. bma.org.uk (accessed 8.11.2020).

Jakab, Z. (2011) Available at: https://www.euro.who.int/__data/assets/pdf_file/0010/135586/RD_speech_Economist_20110317.pdf (accessed 16.10.2020).

Kings Fund, UK (2018). Closing the gap on BME representation in NHS leadership: not rocket science by Mandip Randhawa. Available at: https://www.kingsfund.org.uk/blog/2018/03/bme-representation-nhs-leadership (accessed 21.03.2021).

Kings Fund, UK (2019). We're here and you're there': lived experiences of ethnic minority staff in the NHS by Shilpa Ross. Available at: https://www.kingsfund.org.uk/blog/2019/11/lived-experiences-ethnic-minority-staff-nhs (accessed 21.03.2021).

NHS Digital (2017–2018) Data on written complaints in the NHS.

NHS England (2018) *National NHS Staff Survey*. Available at: https://www.nhsstaffsurveys.com/Page/1101/Past-Results/Staff-Survey-2018-Detailed-Spreadsheets/ (accessed 10.11.2020).

Puddester, D., Flynn, L. and Cohen, J. J. (eds.) (2009) *CanMEDS Physician Health Guide: A Practical Handbook for Physician Health and Well-being*. The Royal College of Physicians and Surgeons of Canada, Canada.

Riskin, A., Erez, A., Foulk, T. A., *et al.* (2015) The impact of rudeness on medical team performance: a randomized trial. *Pediatrics*, **136** (3), 487–495. DOI: 10.1542/peds.2015-1385. Epub 2015 Aug 10. PMID: 26260718.

Royal College of Nursing (2020) *BAME Nursing Staff Experience Greatest PPE Shortages Despite Risk Warnings* (accessed 8.11.2020).

Thomas, C. and Quilter-Pinner, H. (2020) *Care Fit for Carers: Ensuring the Safety and Welfare of NHS and Social Care Workers During and After Covid-19*. Institute for Public Policy Research, London, UK. Available at: https://www.ippr.org/research/publications/care-fit-for-carers (accessed 11.01.2021).

CHAPTER 2

Emotional Impact of Working in Healthcare

Lynn Musto[1] and Julie Carlson[2]

[1] School of Nursing, Trinity Western University, British Columbia, Canada
[2] Fraser Developmental Clinic, British Columbia, Canada

OVERVIEW

- Many health professional–patient interactions are complex. There will inevitably be an emotional impact on practitioners of providing care.
- Emotional impacts of care range from the positive – joy, compassion and engagement – to negative ones – anger, frustration and hopelessness.
- Negative emotional impacts can result in burnout and moral injury.
- Working in healthcare has positive effects on practitioners, including affirmation, a sense of competence, job satisfaction and motivation.
- Authentic relationships with patients protect professionals against some negative costs of caring.
- Practitioners need to develop self-awareness and coping strategies to manage the stresses of healthcare work.

Introduction

Providing care to others has an emotional impact on practitioners because it requires them to extend themselves to another, or many others, every day. With the complexity of treating illness, the emotional impact sits on a spectrum which shifts back and forth between the positive and negative and is dependent on the dynamic nature of the context of treatment. Ideally, practitioners have the time and resources to attend fully to the care required by their patients. This is often not the case in our healthcare systems.

There is increasing awareness of *negative* emotional impacts on practitioners. Burnout, moral distress and vicarious trauma may lead practitioners to emotionally disengage from patients, colleagues and the profession. While disengagement may be a helpful strategy in the short-term for addressing the feeling of being overwhelmed, emotional disengagement contributes also to decreased patient satisfaction and overall health outcomes, increased medical errors and provider dissatisfaction with the profession. While

focusing on alleviating the negative emotional impact of caring is understandable, this approach does obscure the positive emotional impact of caring for others, including the joy and deep satisfaction derived from helping others. Increasingly, healthcare professions and organisations are drawing on the concept of resilience to develop support for practitioners.

The development of resilience is a dynamic process of adaptation in response to challenging, even traumatic experiences. Resilience is a skill developed as practitioners work in healthcare organisations providing patient care.

In this chapter, we discuss a range of emotional consequences resulting from extending oneself on behalf of another. We begin with an outline of the negative emotional impacts of caring for others and discuss the topics of burnout, compassion fatigue, moral distress and vicarious trauma. Thereafter, we consider positive emotional impacts of caring for others and examine the role of empathy and compassion as protective factors against the negative emotional consequences of caring. We conclude with strategies for individuals and organisations directed at reducing the harmful consequences resulting from the negative emotional impact of caring.

The cost of caring

What happens when the emotional content of working with patients combined with systemic pressures become too much? Or when work-life stress coincides with events happening in the practitioner's non-work life? Generally, practitioners enter their profession eager do a good job. Often, we enter our profession believing we have the resources to maintain our mental, emotional and physical health. The result is twofold: (1) we often start working believing burnout is something that happens only to others; and (2) we don't have adequate resources for self-restoration when we become overwhelmed by the needs of our patients. We should ask not what we ought to do *if* we experience the negative consequences of caring, but what we ought to do *when* we experience them.

ABC of Clinical Resilience, First Edition. Edited by Anna Frain, Sue Murphy, and John Frain.
© 2021 John Wiley & Sons Ltd. Published 2021 by John Wiley & Sons Ltd.

Box 2.1 **Definition of terms.**

Concept	Definition
Burnout	Burnout is a psychological syndrome of emotional exhaustion, depersonalisation and reduced personal accomplishment that can occur among individuals who work with other people in some capacity. A key aspect of burnout syndrome is increased feelings of emotional exhaustion, depersonalisation and reduced personal accomplishment (Maslach *et al.*, 1996).
Compassion fatigue	A state of exhaustion and dysfunction – biologically, psychologically and socially – as a result of prolonged exposure to compassion stress and all that it evokes (Figley, 1995).
Moral distress	Moral distress arises when one knows the right thing to do, but institutional constraints make it nearly impossible to pursue the right course of action (Jameton, 1984).
Vicarious trauma	Vicarious trauma is the transformation in the inner experience of the therapist that comes about as a result of empathetic engagement with clients' trauma (Pearlman and Saakvitne, 1995).

Sources: Maslach *et al.* (1996); Figley (1995); Jameton (1984); Pearlman and Saakvitne (1995).

Box 2.2 **The cost of caring.**

Dr Fay, a paediatrician, is going through a complicated divorce. The hospital paediatric ward she has worked on for the past five years has recently begun treating palliative patients. Dr Fay knows that she will need to increase her strategies to manage stress.

Important to this question is the interconnection between our professional and home lives. We hear about the importance of work–life balance, but achieving, and then maintaining, such balance is tenuous. Stressful events in either area of our life will influence our ability to manage all areas of our life. Balance between both areas of life is not easy. Instead, we need to think about developing resources in our life that will sustain us during times of high stress.

Burnout

There has been increasing prevalence of burnout over the past few decades in the general population and specifically in the helping fields. A survey by the Canadian Medical Association (2018) found that, on average, 30% of physicians experienced burnout (Canadian Medical Association, 2018). Dyrbye *et al.* (2017) found that more than half the physicians in the US experienced high rates of burnout, especially those working on the frontlines of care.

Burnout is comprised of three dimensions: overwhelming exhaustion, cynicism and detachment from your job, and a sense of being ineffective in your work (Wagaman *et al.*, 2015). Burnout has been linked to emotional, psychological and physiological consequences for the practitioner; an increase in medical errors; and significant economic cost to healthcare organisations due to increased employee turnover (Bagnall *et al.*, 2016; Reith, 2018).

Moral distress

Moral distress arises in situations where a practitioner believes they are compromised as a moral agent in the context of practicing according to their professional standards and values (Varcoe *et al.*, 2012). The experience of moral distress crosses all disciplines, although the causes of moral distress may differ. Constraints on a practitioner's ability to practice in alignment with their standards of practice or professional values are embedded in the workplace context in the form of policies, limited resources or common practices that violate values of personhood, dignity and respect. The physical, emotional and psychological effects of moral distress (headaches, diarrhoea, disturbed sleep, anger, frustration, anxiety, a sense of powerlessness, self-blame and self-criticism) activate individual protective mechanisms, leading to moral residue or moral disengagement (Rodney *et al.*, 2013).

Compassion fatigue

Healthcare practitioners experience compassion fatigue due to ongoing exposure to the suffering of others (Perry, 2008). Figley (1995) considered compassion fatigue a form of burnout. However, he now argues that compassion fatigue is *secondary traumatic stress* (STS) for which significant healthy coping strategies are needed (Ludick and Figley, 2017). Pathways to experiencing compassion fatigue include exposure to suffering and having empathetic concern for those in our care. Ludick and Figley (2017) have developed a *compassion fatigue resilience model* to explain the development of

Box 2.3 **Case study 1 – moral distress.**

Carmen, a psychiatric nurse, was working in the emergency department. One evening, a woman, Kate, came into the emergency department looking for help. Kate explained that her husband of 30 years had left her several months ago. She was feeling increasingly isolated and lonely; while she was not actively suicidal, she did not know if she could keep herself safe. The emergency department physician assessed Kate and wrote orders for her to be admitted to the hospital as an involuntary patient.

Carmen experienced moral distress as she believed this was a disproportionate and non-therapeutic response as Kate was not actively suicidal and was not a flight risk. Carmen was also aware of the policy which stated that all involuntary patients admitted to the emergency department must be placed in a locked cell with nothing but hospital pyjamas. She believed this was not a therapeutic response and could lead to Kate feeling further isolated and potentially lose trust in the ability of healthcare practitioners to be helpful. Carmen's attempts to advocate for a less restrictive response were rebuffed, and she was ordered to follow hospital policy.

compassion fatigue and provide ideas for developing emotional hardiness and resilience in the face of others' suffering. The first assumptions of the model are that 'STS is a highly complex and often unavoidable experience. . .' (p. 113). Ludick and Figley identify four factors – self-care, detachment (self–other boundary awareness), satisfaction and social support – that require ongoing cultivation. Each offers a pathway for developing resilience as practitioners respond to the emotional needs of patients.

Vicarious trauma

Vicarious trauma occurs when the internal world of the practitioner is negatively transformed through empathetic engagement with individuals who have experienced violence (Pearlman and Saakvitne, 1995; Tabor, 2011). Vicarious trauma has also been referred to as *secondary traumatic stress* and has a presentation that overlaps with compassion fatigue, burnout and disorders that may result from caring. Vicarious trauma has a lasting impact on practitioners, affecting their overall sense of self-identity, worldview and spirituality (Pearlman and Saakvitne, 1995).

Burnout, compassion fatigue, moral distress and vicarious trauma, while distinct experiences, share commonalities such as contributing factors; activation of the stress response and protective mechanisms; and consequences. They also share pathways with empathy and compassion. The pathways for empathy and compassion can lead to joy and satisfaction or negative emotional experiences.

Effects of erosion of empathy, compassion and disengagement

Empathy contributes to the development of the therapeutic relationship, better patient outcomes and higher levels of compassion satisfaction. It may also lead to feeling overwhelmed by the difficult emotions of patients, activating protective mechanisms such as avoidance and disengagement. With emotional and relational disengagement, practitioners carry out the functions of their job without consideration for the emotional experience of others. Behaviours range from a lack of curiosity about patients or colleagues (simply going through the motions of caring – 'box tick-

Box 2.4 **Example 1 of disengagement.**

Bill was a 60-year-old man who arrived in the hospital for a colonoscopy. Bill was anxious about the hospital procedure and worried about the potential results due to a family history of colon cancer. The nurse assigned to Bill for the procedure was straightforward in her presentation of directions, information and her assistance in preparing him for the procedure. Bill noted that the nurse seemed efficient in doing her job, and almost 'robotic'. The nurse did not seem to notice Bill's anxiety and did not offer any compassion or direct reassurance. This nurse presented as disengaged from the human emotions and experiences associated with receiving healthcare, and the disengagement was acutely felt by the patient at a time when engagement would have been likely to decrease the patient's stress level.

Box 2.5 **Example 2 of disengagement.**

Candace had been teaching clients skills to manage mental health symptoms in the local community mental health centre for the past 10 years. Candace worked to develop a therapeutic relationship with her clients, so that she could individualise her teachings and support to fit the client's needs. A year ago, the health authorities decided to standardise all mental healthcare services provided in the community. A 12-week manualised cognitive behavioural training (CBT) course was created that was to be taught in a group setting in all mental health settings in the community. The changes were made so that more clients could be serviced at the centre. The result was that Candace's case load increased as her ability to provide individualised care decreased. Initially, Candace took a wait-and-see attitude about manualised CBT, but she currently feels disconnected from her teaching and the clients as she is simply going through the motions. She does not know how the clients are actually doing, or if the group classes are an effective teaching method, since Candace does not receive any feedback from the health authority.

ing') to a complete disregard for patients and colleagues. Emotional disengagement contributes to patient dissatisfaction and practitioner disenchantment with the care provided.

Disengagement

Various elements contribute to the range of emotional experiences described in the preceding text. Some elements relate to the context of work, such as the increasing acuity of patients and workload, and organisational push for efficiencies. Other factors are interpersonal (e.g., professional or peer support, or a toxic work environment) or intrapersonal (individual exposure to trauma). Most often, it is a combination of external, interpersonal and intrapersonal elements, coming together at a particular moment in time, that undo us. The negative emotional impact of empathy and compassion, along with expectations of care, contributes to the burden experienced by practitioners leading to emotional disengagement.

Media reports on healthcare

Media reports may also have an emotional impact on healthcare practitioners' perspectives on their profession and their work environment. Practitioners – including nurses, physicians, pharmacists and paramedics – are listed near the top in surveys of 'most-trusted' professions. However, individual practitioners may act in ways that violate standards of practice, code of ethics or both. Infamous examples include Elizabeth Wettlaufer or Niels Högel, nurses who abused their position of power inflicting significant harm (and death) to their patients. Media reports sensationalise these stories with headlines about nurse 'serial killers'. Stories about abuse of power, while very distressing, can be attributed to a deeply flawed or disturbed individual, and do not necessarily reflect negatively on a healthcare profession. However, other situations, such as pervasive abuse of patients or poor care contributing to premature death, can reflect badly on health professionals in general.

In the United Kingdom, the Mid Staffordshire Public Health Inquiry examined the appalling conditions and substandard (and, at times, inhumane) hospital care that patients received locally. In published findings, there was a pervasive sentiment that 'certain persons, mostly healthcare professionals (HCPs) knowingly may have been a part of, or turned a blind eye to, these troubling allegations' (Coleman, 2014). This sentiment taints all practitioners as self-serving, contributing to a decreased sense of pride and worth in their chosen profession.

Conversely, not all media reports about healthcare are negative. In fact, public support and media coverage for healthcare practitioners during the COVID-19 pandemic have been overwhelmingly positive. Nightly public applause that celebrates practitioners serves as a reminder of the contribution they make to the lives of others.

The joy of practice

Medical practitioners enter their profession desirous of having positive impacts on their patients. Feelings from helping others have a reciprocal positive effect on the practitioners. Empathy and compassion are foundational to developing genuine relationships with those in our care. Genuine human connection between the practitioner and the patient is a vital part of our work and contributes to an increased sense of purpose and meaning, inoculating practitioners against the occupational hazards of negative emotions (Wagaman *et al.*, 2015).

Compassion satisfaction

Compassion satisfaction is the pleasure experienced from doing our work well (Stamm, 2005). The concept arose from research on compassion fatigue exploring protective factors against burnout and compassion fatigue. Sacco and Copel (2018) defined it as 'the pleasure, purpose, and gratification received by professional caregivers through their contributions to the well-being of patients and their families' (p. 78). Their work involved concept analysis of compassion satisfaction in nursing and outlined antecedents, characteristics and consequences of compassion satisfaction (Figure 2.1). Healthcare

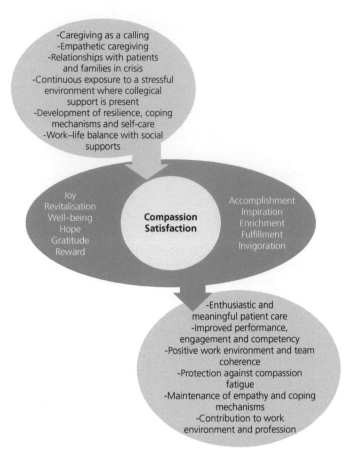

Figure 2.1 Conceptual model of compassion satisfaction. Source: Sacco and Copel (2018). © 2018, John Wiley & Sons.

Box 2.6 **Joy of practice – case history.**

Kyle, a 16-year-old adolescent admitted to a psychiatric unit, was struggling with mental health issues as well as unstable housing that contributed to his mental health issues. Kyle recognised his need for specialised housing that could support him as he learned how to address his mental health needs. Members of his mental health team spent a significant amount of time supporting Kyle in developing a plan so he could advocate for himself in having needs met. In the end, Kyle was discharged to an environment that would foster the best outcome for him. While this was a great discharge and new beginning for Kyle, it also had a positive impact on members of the healthcare team who had spent time reviewing drafts of letters Kyle wrote and role-playing discussions because they witnessed how their clinical efforts made a tangible difference in Kyle's life. As a longer-term consequence, team members also had a template for how to support adolescents in the future who confronted similar situations.

Box 2.7 **Compassion satisfaction vignette.**

Ms. S is a 55-year-old woman who presented for chronic pain care. She had diagnoses of fibromyalgia, anxiety and depression in addition to significant mobility issues that were of unidentified origin. Ms. S had a long history of presenting to emergency departments with pain issues. In a consultation, Ms. S initially presented as guarded, focused on medication and interventional medicine. She also had a long history of not following through with the recommended community services. Ms. S was encouraged to have sessions with allied health within the pain clinic in addition to her primary doctor. These sessions were initially short, and the focus was on relationship building utilising trauma-informed care principles. Over time, Ms. S was able to disclose an extensive history of interpersonal trauma. As she built trust with the practitioner, she became willing to consider trying various approaches to addressing her chronic pain and mental health issues that she was previously unable/unwilling to try, including agreeing to involvement with a community mental health team. Her pain medication dose was decreased, and her presentations to the emergency department became minimal. Ms. S commented to staff in the pain clinic that she did not feel judged within the clinic and felt like the staff believed in her.

Genuine human connection with this woman created a shift in how practitioners interacted with her and improved her engagement with the healthcare system. Ms. S's overall functioning showed improvement, and this was a rewarding experience for the healthcare team as they recognised their contribution.

Box 2.8 **Compassion satisfaction vignette.**

Emily was a 5-year-old girl whose father was hospitalised for a short period and then died unexpectedly on the ward. Emily's mother was distraught and indicated that she felt unprepared to support her daughter in this situation. Hospital nursing and social work staff spent time with Emily. They explained to Emily what had happened to her father, supported her to draw a goodbye card and took her to say goodbye to her father. Although the loss of her father was a tragic event, staff went above and beyond to support her. The staff involved had a genuine emotional connection and felt that this was a meaningful interaction that significantly impacted this child's experience.

Box 2.9 **Case study – self-awareness.**

Patrick was a physiotherapist who received a referral to see an elderly male patient post-stroke. The patient would become angry at times and tearful at other times. He spoke about his changes in function, and his worry that he was not improving quickly enough. Patrick felt empathy and compassion for this patient's frustration, worry, grief and sadness. Patrick's own father had experienced a stroke. Patrick knew that his own emotions (sadness and worry) regarding his father's stroke and the resulting changes in his father's health/functioning was a trigger for him and may impact how he responded to this patient. Patrick monitored his own emotional state while working with this patient and kept a high awareness on his own emotional boundaries (his emotions vs the patient's emotions). Patrick ensured that he elicited the patient's emotions and perspectives and reminded himself that this patient had his personal experiences surrounding the stroke (different from Patrick's father). Patrick used his coping strategies, such as talking to a co-worker and watching comedy clips on his break, to regulate his emotions when the empathy he felt for this patient became distressing for him.

includes helping a patient achieve better health outcomes or move towards their identified health goals; assisting a client in overcoming or learning to live with a chronic illness; decreasing pain; alleviating suffering; or promoting growth and independence. When healthcare practitioners are successful in these endeavours, they experience a sense of achievement and well-being.

Compassion satisfaction motivates and inspires practitioners in their caring role. It reflects the mutual benefit of the helping relationship, whereby patients experience being cared for and practitioners experience affirmation of purpose.

Empathy

Our understanding of empathy continues to evolve with discoveries from neuroscience. We appreciate how fostering empathy in professional relationships supports better health outcomes for patients, and resiliency in practitioners. Empathy comprises both emotional and cognitive components that help practitioners connect with patients' emotional experience (building therapeutic connection). The emotional components are a common focus (understanding, feeling and resonating with the affective states of another person). The cognitive components are crucial to establishing interpersonal boundaries between practitioner and patient.

The cognitive components of empathy include self–other differentiation, perspective-taking and emotion regulation to prevent becoming overwhelmed by the patient's suffering (Decety and Ickes, 2009). When healthcare practitioners become overwhelmed by patients' suffering, protective responses are activated, causing the practitioner to create distance between themselves and the patient. Engaging these cognitive components helps the practitioner maintain 'self–other' awareness, recognising that it is the patient who is suffering. The practitioner remains emotionally connected to the patient without becoming overwhelmed by their emotional state.

Reducing risk and burnout

Interventions to support resiliency need to be directed at both the individual and organisational level, with resources for healthcare practitioners to sustain themselves while building resiliency.

a) Engagement in authentic relationship with patients is a protective factor against the negative costs of caring. Authentic relationships

Box 2.10 **Effect of clinician empathy on patient's recovery from illness.**

Rakel *et al*. (2011) looked at the role of empathy in medical consultations to cold outcomes in a randomised controlled trial.

The authors looked at patient–practitioner interactions, especially the use of empathy (one 'dose' of empathy). The authors assessed the patient's experience of empathy in their consultation using a consultation and relational empathy (CARE) measure. Interleukin 8 (IL8) and neutrophil counts were obtained from nasal wash at baseline and 48 h later.

Patients who perceived the clinician as empathetic (on the CARE measure) reported a shorter duration and severity of the cold. This was corroborated with symptom reports and the IL8 and neutrophil counts. Those who experienced higher perceived empathy got better a full day earlier.

Source: Based on Rakel *et al*. (2011).

(empathy, presence, noting common humanity) create the conditions for compassion satisfaction and effectiveness in practice. Perry (2008) refers to these relational moments as *moments of connection*, making moments matter and energising moments. The nurses in Perry's study (2008) noted that engagement in meaningful human encounters in patient care was experienced as a 'privilege' and a 'gift'. Nurses valued these relationships and relished the opportunity make a difference in the lives of their patients.

Connecting with another human in a state of attunement (empathy) invokes a neurobiological process whereby both parties become more emotionally regulated (Siegel, 2010). It is also crucial that healthcare workers have the self-awareness and strategies to modulate empathy and compassion (Lown, 2016). It is important to use both cognitive strategies and strategies aimed to directly reduce the bodily stress response.

Box 2.11 **Modulators of empathy and compassion.**

- The ability to focus one's attention to recognise, elicit and accurately interpret expressions of emotion
- The ability to listen
- The ability to imagine another's perspective
- The strength of situational empathetic concern
- Non-judgmental positive valuation of others
- Awareness of one's own emotions and subconscious affective biases and triggers
- 'Self–other' boundary awareness
- The ability to regulate one's emotions
- Effective communication skills for use with patients, families, colleagues
- Clinician's own well-being, including self-care and social support

Source: Modified from Lown (2016).

Box 2.12 **Self-care case study.**

Jennifer was a social worker running an educational group for patients with chronic conditions in an inner-city health clinic. The group was comprised of patients living in marginalised conditions and facing many social stressors. Patients often spoke about their past traumatic experiences and current difficult life circumstances. Jennifer knew that the magnitude of the stress and trauma in this patient population had the potential to have a negative impact on her (including a cumulative effect). Jennifer often spent a few moments doing deep breathing during the group break time. Jennifer also made it a regular purposeful practice, when driving home after group sessions, to sing along to her favourite songs in the car. Jennifer knew from experience that this activity assisted her to decrease her stress response and regulate her emotions. Jennifer also knew that this was a strategy she could commit to using in her busy schedule before arriving home to her family.

---

b) Several cognitive strategies assist practitioners to modulate the experience of empathy and compassion for their patients. Self-awareness of one's own emotions and triggers is crucial. Emotional boundaries are necessary and have a positive impact in reducing burnout (Wagaman *et al.*, 2015). Espeland (2006 cited in Perry, 2008) reported that an individual healthcare practitioner's attitude may help prevent compassion fatigue and burnout. This includes a positive attitude, positive energy and an appropriate sense of humour regarding healthcare work. Core personal and professional values underpin attitude, and maintaining an explicit focus on these values is helpful (Perry, 2008).

Cognitive reappraisal (attaching different meanings to an experience) assists the practitioner in regulating emotions (Lown, 2016). For example, in patients with complex and chronic health issues, shifting the practitioner's views of success away from recovery and towards increases in functionality, quality of life or a patient's ability to take positive steps for themselves can assist with healthcare practitioner's ability to attune and be present with the emotional experience of the patient.

c) Personal coping strategies are an integral piece in building resilience as an engaged and compassionate practitioner. Practitioners need to attend to self-care to remain regulated and attune and engage with patients. Some of the regulatory bodies consider effective self-care a professional obligation and include self-care in their standards of practice (e.g., Canadian Code of Ethics for Psychology and Professional Standards for Psychiatric Nurses in British Columbia, Canada).

Most healthcare professionals can likely cite some 'self-care' strategies. It is important that practitioners personalise strategies and do so prior to facing a highly stressful incident at their workplace. Often, practitioners do not have a meaningful plan for self-care until it is too late. Personalising means trying strategies and appraising whether they result in a personal reduction in stress, increase in a sense of well-being and/or invoke the feeling of joy. Possibilities for self-care are endless (including exercise, hobbies, connection with friends/family, relaxation exercises, etc.). However, the value lies in the personal response to the activity.

Healthcare practitioners need immediate strategies that they can use to address their stress response. These include breathing exercises and grounding exercises (activities intended to bring your attention to your body in the present moment to reduce nervous system activity). Larger activities (meaningful to the practitioner, such as hobbies, social groups or exercise) that are engaged in regularly and readily available in times of stress are also necessary.

Mindfulness practices may decrease stress in the short term and, with regular practice, create brain changes in areas that process emotions and manage stress. Investing time in these practices is likely to have a positive impact on practitioner resiliency (Raab, 2014). Self-compassion is a related concept involving self-acceptance, non-judgement and kindness to oneself. Self-compassion skills can be taught and learned. Practicing self-compassion leads to more compassion satisfaction and less likelihood of experiencing compassion fatigue. People with skills in self-compassion are more likely to recognise the emotional difficulty of providing care to those who are suffering and then care for their own emotional needs, such as taking time off or getting more sleep (Neff, 2011).

Conclusions

Provision of compassionate, empathetic care is a two-sided coin. Extending compassion and empathy to those in our care helps ground practitioners in a deep sense of meaning and purpose in their professional life. Empathetic engagement also exposes practitioners to risks of burnout, compassion fatigue, moral distress and vicarious trauma. In the face of increasing institutional pressures and the suffering of others, our protective mechanisms activate the desire to avoid and disengage. These can be important responses in the short-term but are detrimental to everyone involved in caring. Developing resilience using effective, individualised self-care strategies is essential for a sustained and meaningful career in the healthcare field. The question to ask at the beginning of our career is not 'if' but 'when' we will need these strategies.

Further reading/resources

Bagnall, A., Jones, R., Akter, H. and Woodall, J.R. (2016) *Interventions to Prevent Burnout in High Risk Individuals: Evidence Review*. Public Health England, London, UK.

Canadian Medical Association (2018) *CMA National Physician Health Survey: A National Snapshot*. Canadian Medical Association, Ottawa, ON.

Coleman, A. (2014) Post mid-Staffordshire inquiries reaction, in and about the National Health Service (NHS), England. The missing pieces: Organizational, care and virtue ethics perspectives. *International Journal of Clinical Medicine*, **5** (16), 1009–1015.

Decety, J. and Ickes, W. (eds) (2009) *The Social Neuroscience of Empathy*. MIT Press, Cambridge, MA.

Dyrbye, L.N., Shanafelt, T.D., Sinsky, C. A. *et al.* (2017) Burnout among health care professionals: A call to explore and address this underrecognized threat to safe, high-quality care. Discussion Paper, *National Academy of Medicine*, Washington DC.

Espeland, K. (2006) Overcoming burnout: how to revitalize your career. *The Journal of Continuing Education in Nursing*, **37** (4), 178–184.

Figley, C.R. (1995) Compassion fatigue: toward a new understanding of the costs of caring, in *Secondary Traumatic Stress: Self-care Issues for Clinicians, Researchers, and Educators* (ed B.H. Stamm, pp. 3–28). The Sidran Press, Lutherville, MD.

Jameton, A. (1984) *Nursing Practice: The Ethical Issues*. Prentice-Hall, Englewood Cliffs, N.J.

Lown, B.A. (2016) A social neuroscience-informed model for teaching and practicing compassion in health care. *Medical Education*, **50** (3), 332–342.

Ludick, M. and Figley, C.R. (2017) Toward a mechanism for secondary trauma induction and reduction: reimagining a theory of secondary traumatic stress. *Traumatology*, **23** (1), 112.

Maslach, C., Jackson, S.E., Leiter, M.P. *et al.* (1996) *Maslach Burnout Inventory*, 3rd edition manual. *CPP Inc*, Mountain View, CA.

Neff, K. (2011) *The Proven Power of Being Kind to Yourself: Self-compassion* (pp. 192–193). Harper Collin, New York, NY.

Pearlman, L.A. and Saakvitne, K.W. (1995) *Trauma and the Therapist: Countertransference and Vicarious Traumatization in Psychotherapy with Incest Survivors*. WW Norton & Company, New York.

Perry, B. (2008) Why exemplary oncology nurses seem to avoid compassion fatigue. *Canadian Oncology Nursing Journal*, **18** (2), 87–92.

Raab, K. (2014) Mindfulness, self-compassion, and empathy among health care professionals: a review of the literature. *Journal of Health Care Chaplaincy*, **20** (3), 95–108.

Rakel, D., Barrett, B., Zhang, Z. *et al.* (2011). Perception of empathy in the therapeutic encounter: effects on the common cold. *Patient education and Counseling*, **85** (3), 390–397.

Reith, T.P. (2018) Burnout in United States Healthcare Professionals: a narrative review. *Cureus*, **10** (12), e3681.

Rodney, P. et al. (2013) *Toward a Moral Horizon: Nursing Ethics for Leadership and Practice* (pp. 160–187), Pearson Education, Canada.

Sacco, T.L. and Copel, L.C. (2018) Compassion satisfaction: a concept analysis in nursing. *Nursing Forum*, **53** (1), 76–83. https://doi.org/10.1111/nuf.12213

Siegel, D.J. (2010). *The Mindful Therapist: A Clinician's Guide to Mindsight and Neural Integration (Norton Series on Interpersonal Neurobiology)*. WW Norton & Company, New York, NY.

Stamm, B.H. (2005) *The ProQUAL Manual*. Sidran Press, Pocatello, ID.

Tabor, P.D. (2011) Vicarious traumatization: Concept analysis. *Journal of Forensic Nursing*, **7** (4), 203–208.

Varcoe, C., Pauly, B., Webster, G.C. and Storch, J.L. (2012) Moral distress: tensions as springboards for action. *HEC Forum*, **24** (1), 51–62.

Wagaman, M.A., Geiger, J.M., Shockley, C. and Segal, E.A. (2015) The role of empathy in burnout, compassion satisfaction, and secondary traumatic stress among social workers. *Social Work*, **60** (3), 201–209.

CHAPTER 3

Resilience and Cognitive Performance

John Frain

Division of Medical Sciences and Graduate Entry Medicine, University of Nottingham, UK

OVERVIEW

- The ability to diagnose and appropriately treat patients is the most critical of the healthcare professional's skills.
- Clinical decision-making requires optimal cognitive function, which is dependent on physiological well-being.
- The cognitive process of clinical decision-making is prone to inherent biases and contextual factors such as clinician anxiety, uncertainty and the effects of psychosocial stress.
- Healthcare organisations should support clinicians' cognitive performance by ensuring healthcare professionals' hierarchy of needs is met and maintained.
- Organisations not addressing the cognitive well-being of healthcare professionals are placing patients at risk of harm.
- Health professional training programmes should address students' response to anxiety and uncertainty so that they become cognitively self-aware.

Introduction

To the layperson, it inevitably appears that 'there must be something they can do' – that healthcare is more definitive than is the reality. Many new students, on entering their chosen discipline, struggle with this concept. There must be one question, one physical sign, one lab or imaging test which will give a definitive answer to a clinical problem – 'yes' or 'no', 'positive' or 'negative'. Discovery of the sometimes ambiguous and uncertain nature of practice is something with which all clinicians must contend in their development. Ability to tolerate this uncertainty has a profound impact on clinical practice and patient care (Iannello *et al.*, 2017). Through the learning process, students realise that every aspect of healthcare is affected by uncertainty and ambiguity. The sources of this uncertainty include the following:

- Limited medical knowledge for:
  - Making a diagnosis
  - Choosing a treatment

- Unpredictability or unfamiliarity with the natural history of a patient's disease
- Variability of patients' responses to treatment

The ability to cope with uncertainty and ambiguity is a required competence of clinicians. It is an aspect of clinical reasoning and has been described as 'cognitive flexibility' (Nijstad *et al.*, 2010). Uncertainty is perceived invariably by the individual as a threat – possible harm to the patient, but also harm to the clinician as the 'second victim' of a mistake (see Chapter 4). Higher cognitive ability depends on working memory, attention span and control processes such as inhibition, shifting attention, updating and maintenance. Cognitive function is affected by increasing age and stress. We do not yet fully understand the anatomy and physiology of the pathways by which these functions are mediated. However, there is unambiguous evidence that stress and resilience, cardiovascular and cognitive function are interrelated and interdependent. In this chapter, we will discuss the impact of resilience on cognitive performance. It has implications for patient safety.

Clinical reasoning

The thinking and decision-making processes associated with practice are referred to as *clinical reasoning*, which is a complex task requiring the interpretation of many data streams and subject to many influences. Dual process theory describes the process of analysing a patient's presentation and diagnosis (Norman and Eva, 2010) (Table 3.1). Experimental evidence supports the anatomical and physiological existence of two reasoning systems. Type 1 thinking is associated with the ventral medial prefrontal cortex, and Type 2 with the right inferior prefrontal cortex. The two sites may have differing glucose requirements (Kern, 2008) – a simple fact illustrative of the need for regular meal breaks to facilitate good decision-making during shifts.

Referred to as *Type 1* and *Type 2 thinking*, students and junior practitioners will tend to take a more deliberate and stepwise (Type 2) approach to diagnosis (Croskerry, 2009). With the accumulation of

---

experience in seeing patients ('illness scripts'), faster, more intuitive (Type 1) thinking is possible (Table 3.1). This is an oversimplification. In reality, the expert clinician oscillates between Type 1 and Type 2, depending on the complexity of the patient's problem. Similarly, the reasoning process is far more complicated than simply two types of thinking (Figure 3.1).

Despite technological advances, diagnosis is still dependent on complete data collection (history and examination) as well as effective cognitive performance in its interpretation. Paradoxically, greater use of technology and the more detailed revelation of the disease process can actually increase uncertainty (e.g., setting the threshold for abnormality in a diagnostic test). Causes of diagnostic error are multifactorial, but human causes include inadequate data collection and faulty reasoning. Both are related to tolerance of ambiguity and uncertainty, and to psychological well-being (Box 3.1).

Biases and contextual factors

Clinical reasoning is subject to potential for cognitive error (bias) (Table 3.2). It takes place within the context of the workplace environment, the patient's and professional's personal perspectives and the patient–professional relationship. Many diagnostic errors are associated with faulty clinical reasoning. Rates are higher in internal

Table 3.1 Characteristics of Type 1 and Type 2 thinking.

Type 1 thinking	Type 2 thinking
• Intuitive, uses mental shortcuts (heuristics) • Automatic, subconscious • Fast, effortless • Low/variable reliability • Vulnerable to error • Highly affected by context • High emotional involvement • Low scientific rigour	• Analytical, systematic • Deliberate, conscious • Slow, effortful • High/consistent reliability • Less prone to error • Less affected by context • Low emotional involvement • High scientific rigour

Source: Cooper and Frain (2017). © 2016, John Wiley & Sons.

> Box 3.1 **Case study: effect of fatigue on clinical performance.**
>
> Saima, an experienced physiotherapist, has been up most of the night due to her 15-month-old baby having a temperature. She is working in ITU the following day. She struggled to manage Mr Singh, a Covid-19 patient, who required intensive chest physiotherapy. She could not understand what was wrong as she had managed it perfectly the previous day.

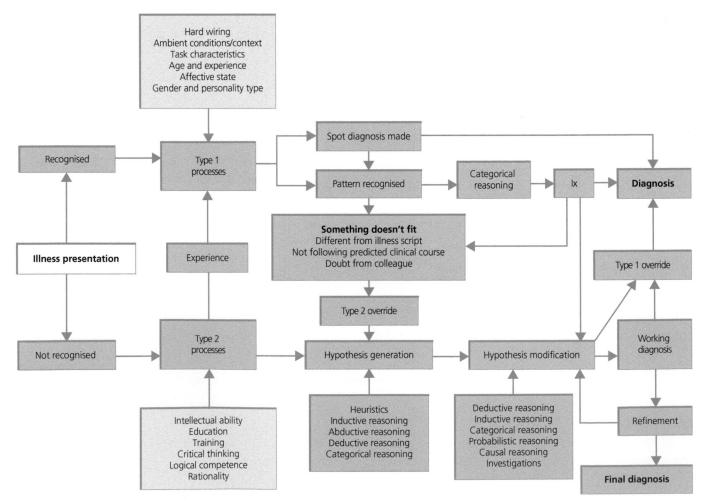

Figure 3.1 A modified universal model of diagnostic reasoning. Source: Cooper and Frain (2017). © 2016, John Wiley & Sons.

Table 3.2 Examples of cognitive errors (bias) in clinical reasoning.

Error	Description
Anchoring	Having latched on to a particular aspect of the initial consultation, we refuse to change our mind about the importance of the aspect.
Confirmation bias	Once we have made an initial diagnosis, we tend to accept evidence which backs our hypothesis and ignore evidence which refutes it.
Premature closure	We make a diagnosis before all the information has been gathered or verified. This involves short-cutting to the final diagnosis stage when we should only be at the hypothesis generation and modification stage.
Search satisficing	Once we have made a diagnosis, we forget that there may be others. We commonly miss second fractures or second poisoning agents.
Posterior probability error	Short-cutting to the patient's usual diagnosis. The patient may have presented with confusion and agitation from alcohol withdrawal many times earlier, but it is wise to check for alternatives, such as pneumonia or subdural haematoma.
Outcome bias	Our desire for a certain outcome alters our judgement (e.g., a surgeon blaming sepsis on pneumonia rather than an anastomotic leak).

Source: Cooper and Frain (2017). © 2016, John Wiley & Sons.

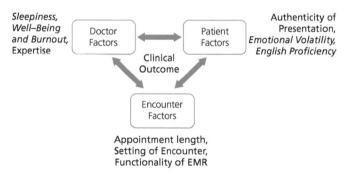

Figure 3.2 Situated cognition as a framework for context within a sample clinical encounter. Clinical outcome is dependent upon complex interactions among all components – the physician, the patient and the encounter. EMR = electronic medical record. Source: McBee *et al.* (2017). Licensed under CC BY 4.0.

medicine, where there is more likely to be complexity and greater uncertainty (van den Berge and Mamede, 2013). The focus of our discussion here is the contextual factors and, in particular, the effect of these on the health professional's care of the patient. This has been referred to as a 'situated cognition' and describes a complex encounter as shaped by the social context of the participants and the environment in which it occurs (Figure 3.2) (McBee *et al.*, 2017). For a more detailed perspective on clinical reasoning, the reader is referred to *ABC of Clinical Reasoning* (Cooper and Frain, 2017).

The highest level of Maslow's pyramid is 'problem solving' (see Chapter 4). Professional self-image in the health disciplines includes successful problem-solving. For example, for a doctor, this includes making the correct diagnosis, while, for a physiotherapist, it may include assisting a patient to feed themselves or to climb the steps to their home. Successful problem-solving is vital for patient safety. For the professional, successful problem-solving contributes to the fulfilment and personal well-being which should come from

Table 3.3 Contextual factors relevant to clinical decision-making and patient safety.

Organisational factors
  Workload
    Inadequate staffing and supervision
  Access to rest breaks, food and drink
  Time pressures
    Impaired information and data gathering
  Disruptions
    Emergencies
    Phone calls
    Staff enquiries
  Access to resources – imaging, equipment
Effects of low tolerance of uncertainty and ambiguity
  Higher referral rates
  Increased use of diagnostic tests
  Anxiety
  Reduced job satisfaction
  More discomfort in dealing with dying patients or complex cases
  Increased dogmatism, rigidity and conformism
Patient factors
  Communicating in a second language
  Emotional volatility
Clinician factors
  Sleep deprivation
Self-rated sleepiness
  Burnout

Source: Adapted from McBee *et al.* (2017).

work. However desirable, it is not a cold, logical process but occurs in the context of human beings helping other human beings. The literature increasingly recognises the impacts of contextual factors and tolerance of uncertainty and ambiguity on clinicians' cognitive function (Table 3.3). The following four categories are identifiable as consequences of contextual factors:

- Emotional reactions
- Behavioural inferences
- Optimising the healthcare professional–patient relationship
- Difficulty with closure of the clinical encounter

Organisational and individual commitment to self-awareness and optimising cognitive performance is in the interests of both clinician and organisational well-being – and essential for patient safety as well. This requires meeting the clinician's hierarchy of needs, which helps in better clinical decision-making (Figure 3.3). Though much attention is paid to study of the cognitive steps of clinical reasoning, optimal reasoning and decision-making is dependent on all the needs in the hierarchy being met. Healthcare institutions understandably consider the impact on patients of errors in clinical decision-making, but sometimes overlook how the system has undermined the cognitive performance of professionals. This begins with organisational culture and leadership. Environments characterised by rudeness (Frost uses the term 'toxic emotions at work'; see Frost, 2003) impair the performance of those working in them. This is seen in the accuracy of diagnostic and procedural tasks, which are more checklist-based, and increases further for those tasks requiring teamwork and communication between individuals (Riskin *et al.*, 2013). Pressure on clinicians against taking water-breaks or being seen by patients while drinking coffee or eating lunch reduces a professional's sense of being

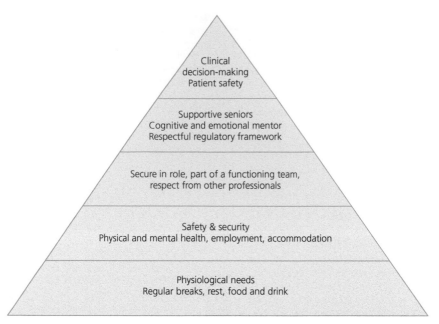

Figure 3.3 Hierarchy of needs for optimal clinical decision-making. Source: Adapted from Maslow's pyramid (Maslow, 1954).

Box 3.2 Case study: limited access to sustenance during shifts.

Alice was working a 12-hour shift in the emergency department. It had been a very busy morning, and she had missed her break due to helping with an unwell patient in Resus. She had not eaten or even had anything to drink since breakfast before coming to work. Going into the office, she fetched a glass of water and returned to her workstation on the unit. As she sat sipping the water and looking at a set of results, she heard a raised voice from one of the senior nurses, 'You are not supposed to eat and drink in the unit'. 'But it is just a glass of water; I missed my break earlier', replied Alice. 'That's not my problem. You are not supposed to eat and drink in the unit. Either go outside or wait until your next break'.

Later, Alice spoke to her friends working in other parts of the hospital. It seemed many of the managers did not like junior doctors to be drinking or eating within sight of patients, since they thought it may create the impression that staff are not prioritising patient care – and unprofessional.

valued and personal well-being (Box 3.2). Unduly hierarchical and/or competitive environments within teams may make clinicians reluctant to seek advice or help from senior staff. Contextual workplace factors allied to the challenge of adapting to the uncertainty and ambiguity inherent to clinical practice can engender a state of perpetual anxiety in clinicians. Consequently, the ability to acquire and apply new knowledge and to internalise the lessons of practice in a manner which develops clinical decision-making is inevitably impaired. Unfortunately, the individual is led to believe the fault lies within themselves more often than the context in which they are being left to work. A consequence is the development of burnout, described in 40–50% of healthcare staff in the United States (Chemali *et al.*, 2019). Burnout predicts increased rates of self-reported medical error.

Burnout and cognitive function

Long-term exposure to stress may affect the autonomic regulation of stress response (see Chapter 5). This affects cardiovascular health and cognitive function. Consequences may include less adaptability and flexibility to stress, as well as altered resilience. Emotional states may be heightened, and this further affects cardiovascular and cognitive health. Work-related stress in middle age is predictive of cognitive decline in older age. Palliative care professionals with higher levels of burnout show alterations in inhibition levels, working memory and decision-making capabilities (Fernandez-Sanchez *et al.*, 2018).

Heart rate variability (HRV) appears related to regulation of the autonomic stress response. It is also linked to prefrontal cortex activity mediated by the vagus nerve linking the brain and the heart. HRV is predictive of cognitive control tasks reliant on the prefrontal cortex. Individuals with higher resting HRV states have greater cognitive flexibility in shifting between tasks (Stenfors *et al.*, 2016). Lower HRV is associated with the onset of symptoms of chronic stress, exhaustion and depression. These conditions are related to impairment of higher cognitive functions, which are required for clinical decision-making. HRV arises from the sympathetic and parasympathetic arms of the autonomic nervous system. Maladaptive states such as chronic stress may lead to imbalance of autonomic regulation and impact cognitive function. This phenomenon has been described in association with psychiatric disease. HRV is sensitive to the needs of sustained attention, concentration and cognitive stress. This may be relevant to the slow, deliberative reasoning (Type 2 thinking) required in complex clinical decision-making. Similarly, better cardiovascular regulation may be associated with improved cognitive control (inhibition, shifting, updating), again relevant for coping with the vagaries of practice and analytical thinking. In addition to the 'thinking-in-the-moment' of patient care, cognitive control is required for reflection on care given, and emotional response to and evaluation of the decision-making after the event (Box 3.3).

Box 3.3 **'Thinking-in-the-moment' and cognitive control.**

Patrick was just coming to the end of busy evening surgery when he was messaged by the practice nurse about a patient who was attending for an asthma review. She had developed a productive cough with green sputum. Patrick agreed to review her and thought the physical examination was normal, with only a few scattered crackles in the chest. He was about to prescribe some antibiotics and steroids for her when he realised that he had not checked her peak flow or oxygen saturation. Both were reduced, putting the patient into a category where she required hospital referral for further assessment. Patrick arranged for this, and the patient was very grateful that he had seen her so promptly.

Driving home, Patrick felt disturbed and a sense of doom or guilt. What if it hadn't occurred to him to look at the remaining vital signs and he had sent the patient home? She could have come to serious harm. He had been feeling very tired by the end of surgery. He found himself waking during the night thinking about it.

The following morning, the incident came up over a coffee with one of his partners, Andrew, who was very reassuring. 'Yes, you almost missed this information, and yes, the patient could have been harmed, but the fact is you didn't. You realised and, because you then checked, the patient received appropriate referral and will be ok'.

Patrick felt relieved to receive this perspective. He realised the benefit of thinking decisions through and reflecting on them, as it could be both a learning point and reassuring that he had acted appropriately. Patrick felt more confident about his actions, though he decided also to include it in his appraisal submission as an example of reflection.

Box 3.4 **The consultant who held my bleep.**

I remember the days when we used to do 48-hour on-calls. I was working in a paediatric unit at the time, and it was extremely busy. Twenty admissions per day was not unusual. As senior house officers, we often got only 2–3 hours of sleep. Our lives were always easier when a particular consultant was on duty. He used to come in for the morning ward round and take a lot of time with the patients and with us, ensuring everything was thoroughly sorted out. Even better than this, he would then take all of our bleeps, so we could go and get to the canteen before it shut and have a proper Sunday lunch.

I've met and worked with many caring people, but I remember him especially fondly as he was so considerate towards us all. We felt part of a team of equals despite the differences in knowledge and experience.

Stress and burnout produce changes in the prefrontal gyri, where analytical thinking occurs. These are identifiable on MRI scans, with burnout particularly affecting the right prefrontal cortex, which is associated with working memory tasks and Type 2 thinking (Durning *et al.*, 2013). Additionally, changes are observable also in the right middle frontal gyrus, an area sensitive to emotionally distressing visual cues, perspective-taking and empathy. Thus, affective changes may change higher cognitive function and contribute to unconscious bias towards patients (Wayne *et al.*, 2011). Such changes are reversible. For example, the study suggested the MRI changes resolved when the requirement to think about a clinical problem was removed ('I feel so much better when I am away from work'). This suggests that the stressors arise from within the workplace, and modification of these stressors may have a beneficial effect on individuals vulnerable to burnout (Box 3.4). Similarly, the individuals themselves can address the effects of stress on their cardiovascular and cognitive functions through measures including regular exercise and reflective practice.

The negativity bias

This describes the tendency to emphasise and remember negative experiences. Much of health professional education is characterised by this approach – 'what did we get right'/'what did we get wrong', rather than 'what did we learn to understand'? Clinicians in every profession tend to perfectionism and competitiveness. Whilst it is clearly in the interest of patients that clinicians strive to know and to do well, it is where this becomes an unforgiving and relentless

culture that the professional is placed at risk of physical, mental and cognitive harm. Paradoxically, however well intentioned, this may be more likely to impair patient safety.

Considering the possible adverse outcomes of a course of action is protective and has a personal and community benefit in preventing harm. However, it can reinforce defensive thinking and practice. The clinician making a wrong diagnosis, when not enabled to reflect on the clinical and contextual factors leading to the error, may instead become inhibited from further development of decision-making skills to avoid further mistakes. Investigation rates, referrals and overdiagnosis may all increase, resulting in job dissatisfaction and, paradoxically, possible patient harm.

Effect of experience

Evidence suggests that clinicians' perception of work-related stress is likely to decrease with experience. Junior clinicians appear more susceptible to burnout and emotional exhaustion (Durning *et al.*, 2013). Recently qualified professionals are particularly susceptible to intolerance of uncertainty and difficulties in developing clinical decision-making skills, leading to doubts about continuing their healthcare career, burnout and leaving the profession. Years of experience and repeated encounters with a range and variety of patient presentations and outcomes may lead to greater self-awareness, confidence and a sense of control in the healthcare environment. This increased cognitive control may make more senior clinicians less susceptible to the effects of burnout. This may arise through automatisation of some aspects of clinical reasoning, resulting in lesser requirement of cognitive resources. However, experienced clinicians remain susceptible to bias and therefore to error (Mamede *et al.*, 2010). In addition, the stress response is both idiosyncratic and variable over time. The senior clinician's cognitive performance may be affected by personal health, caring roles outside work, greater management responsibilities with seniority and involvement in complaints and investigations.

Training needs

From the outset, the uncertain nature of clinical practice should be acknowledged to trainees. It should be disclosed to them that this uncertainty arises both from the limitations of the clinician's

Table 3.4 Strategies for improving tolerance of uncertainty in decision-making.

- Careful data-gathering (history)
- Structured physical examination
- Working within the framework of differential diagnosis
- Considering alternative hypotheses
- Excluding 'must-not-miss' diagnoses
- Using best available evidence
- Re-evaluating the management plan
- Seeking advice from colleagues
- Sharing limitations of knowledge with patient
- Shared decision-making with patient.
- Role-modelling reflection

Source: Based on Iannello *et al.* (2017).

knowledge, particularly in the early years of practice, and from the limitations of the knowledge available to us. Coping with this is a professional competence and includes acquiring good data collection skills as well as optimal reasoning expertise. In addition to discussing the factual and reasoning aspects of patient presentations, a metacognitive approach ('thinking about the thinking') may aid students in recognising the cognitive and emotional impacts on their clinical reasoning (Colombo *et al.*, 2010). This could be addressed by including these factors in the text of vignettes and cases used in teaching clinical reasoning. This reflective approach would enable students to more fully appreciate how contextual factors present during patient encounters may affect their situational awareness, clinical reasoning, and diagnostic accuracy. Reflective reasoning may also address biases and improve diagnostic accuracy (van den Berge and Mamede, 2013). Allied to techniques for maintaining well-being, this may help health professional students and those in training develop strategies for mitigating the effects of burnout and enhancing recovery. Strategies to acknowledge and cope with uncertainty can improve tolerance over time (Table 3.4).

Role-modelling of reflective clinical reasoning by clinical teachers is essential (Kim and Lee, 2018). This could involve:

- Discussing various sources of alternative information about health
- Acknowledging own knowledge gaps
- Being seen to look things up in front of both students and patients
- Displaying empathy to patients and students
- Involving patients and the team in clinical decision-making
- Admitting and reflecting on own biases
- Sharing aspects of personal well-being which have affected clinical work (e.g., a patient complaint or failing an exam)

Conclusions

While cognitive function declines over the lifecycle, junior healthcare professionals are more prone to the cognitive effects of anxiety, psychosocial stress and burnout. Trainees should be taught self-awareness in recognising their own idiosyncratic physiological response to stress and the effect it will have on their cognitive performance and clinical decision-making. Healthcare organisations should ensure that professionals' physical and psychosocial needs are met, which will enable them to problem-solve at their own best level ('to be the best clinician they can be'). In this sense, a 'duty of care' exists on the part of healthcare organisations toward helping clinicians' maintain cognitive well-being. In particular, where correction,

feedback or remediation is needed, it should not involve the destruction of any clinician's physical or mental well-being – nor, when it occurs, should such damage be considered either merely regrettable or acceptable 'collateral damage', given the aims of the organisation overall. To ignore this is to place patients at risk of harm.

Further reading/resources

Chemali, Z., Ezzeddine, F.L., Gelaye, B. *et al.* (2019) Burnout among healthcare providers in the complex environment of the Middle East: a systematic review. *BMC Public Health*, **19**, 1337.

Colombo, B., Iannello, P. and Antonietti, A. (2010) Metacognitive knowledge of decision-making: an explorative study, in *Trends and prospects in metacognitive research* (eds. A. Efklides and P. Misailidi, pp. 445–472). Springer, New York.

Cooper, N. and Frain, J. (2017) *ABC of Clinical Reasoning*. Wiley, Oxford.

Croskerry, P. (2009) A universal model of diagnostic reasoning. *Academic Medicine: Journal of the Association of American Medical Colleges*, **84** (8),1022–1028. DOI: 10.1097/ACM.0b013e3181ace703. PMID: 19638766.

Durning, S.J., Costanzo, M., Artino, A.R. Jr. *et al.* (2013) Functional neuroimaging correlates of burnout among internal medicine residents and faculty members. *Frontiers in Psychiatry*, **4**, 131.

Fernandez-Sanchez, J.C., Perez-Marmol, J.M., Santoz-Ruiz, A.M. *et al.* (2018) Burnout and executive functions in Palliative Care health professionals: influence of burnout on decision making. *Anales del Sistema Sanitario de Navarra*, **41** (2), 171–180.

Frost, P.J. (2003) *Toxic Emotions at Work: How Compassionate Managers Handle Pain and Conflict*. Harvard Business School Press, Boston.

Iannello, P., Mottini, A., Tirelli, S. *et al.* (2017) Ambiguity and uncertainty tolerance, need for cognition, and their association with stress. A study among Italian practicing physicians, *Medical Education Online*, **22**: (1), 1270009. DOI: 10.1080/10872981.2016.1270009.

Kern, S., Oakes, T.R., Stone, C.K. *et al.* (2008) Glucose metabolic changes in the prefrontal cortex are associated with HPA axis response to a psychosocial stressor. *Psychoneuroendocrinology*, **33** (4), 517–529.

Kim, K. and Lee, Y.M. (2018) Understanding uncertainty in medicine: concepts and implications in medical education. *Korean Journal of Medical Education*, **30** (3), 181–188. DOI: 10.3946/kjme.2018.92. Epub 2018 Aug 27. PMID: 30180505; PMCID: PMC6127608.

Mamede, S., van Gog, T., van den Berge, K. *et al.* (2010) Effect of availability bias and reflective reasoning on diagnostic accuracy among internal medicine residents. *JAMA*, **304** (11), 1198–1203.

Maslow, A.H. (1954) *Motivation and Personality*. Harper and Row, New York.

McBee, E., Ratcliffe, T., Picho, K. *et al.* (2017) Contextual factors and clinical reasoning: differences in diagnostic and therapeutic reasoning in board certified versus resident physicians. *BMC Medical Education*, **17** (1), 211.

Nijstad, B., De Dreu, C.K.W., Rietzschel, E.F. and, Baas, M. (2010). The dual pathway to creativity model: Creative ideation as a function of flexibility and persistence. *European Review of Social Psychology*, **21** (1), 34–77.

Norman, G.R. and Eva, K.W. (2010). Diagnostic errors and clinical reasoning. *Medical Education*, **44**, 94–100.

Riskin, A., Erez, A., Foulk, T.A. *et al.* (2013) The impact of rudeness on medical team performance: a randomised trial. *Paediatrics*, **136** (3), 487–495.

Stenfors, C.U., Hanson, L.M., Theorell, T. and Osika, W.S. (2016) Executive cognitive functioning and cardiovascular autonomic regulation in a population-based sample of working adults. *Frontiers in Psychology*, **7**, 1536.

van den Berge, K. and Mamede, S. (2013) Cognitive diagnostic error in medicine. *European Journal of Internal Medicine*, **24**, 525–529.

Wayne, S., Dellmore, D., Serna, L. *et al.* (2011) The association between intolerance of ambiguity and decline in medical students attitudes toward the underserved. *Academic Medicine*, **86** (7), 877–882.

CHAPTER 4

Practising Self-care

Susanne Hewitt[1], Sarah Nicholls[2], and Anna Frain[3]

[1] Emergency Medicine, University Hospitals of Derby & Burton NHS Foundation Trust, UK
[2] Emergency Department, Queens Medical Centre, Nottingham, UK
[3] University of Nottingham, Graduate Entry Medical School, Derby Specialty Training Programme for General Practice, UK

OVERVIEW

- Clinicians tend towards self-criticism, recalling the negative more than success.
- Developing self-awareness and reflective practice is crucial for maintaining resilience and well-being during a career in healthcare and for keeping patients safe.
- Personal needs and solutions change during the career cycle, with identifiable stages requiring different approaches.
- Achieving work–life balance is challenging and our ability to achieve it varies through our careers.
- Personal crises, complaints and negativity have impacts on clinical resilience, which can be recognised and managed.
- The practice of self-care and reflective practice should be integrated with training programmes.

Introduction

'Somehow, we've come to equate success with not needing anyone. Many of us are willing to extend a helping hand, but we're very reluctant to reach out for help when we need it ourselves. It's as if we've divided the world into 'those who offer help' and 'those who need help'. The truth is we are both'.

– Brene Brown

Effectiveness as a clinician requires physical well-being and optimal cognitive performance. This was recognised in ancient times (Box 4.1). Mental and physical abilities naturally decline during a working lifetime. This is balanced by the accumulation of clinical experience ('wisdom'). Related to this is the importance of maintaining our resilience, given the stressful nature of healthcare work. Clinical resilience can develop and accumulate throughout a career. In this chapter, we discuss ways to practise self-care which help both personally and professionally.

Self-aware not self-critical

An effective clinician can identify personal strengths and weaknesses. Finding gaps in knowledge and practical skills facilitates further education and learning to improve clinical performance. Reflection is a useful tool that helps improve confidence, skills and, ultimately, patient safety.

Healthcare professions often attract high achievers who may be naturally self-critical. Negative self-talk can slowly chip away at self-confidence, reinforcing beliefs of being 'not good enough'. This is sometimes referred to as 'imposter syndrome' (see Box 4.2). Professionals can feel they do not fit into their role and will be 'found out' when someone realises they are inferior and unworthy of filling their position. When things go wrong, as they do for everyone, it is important to be self-aware, and not self-critical.

Table 4.1 provides examples to highlight key differences between self-criticism and self-awareness. Appreciating the difference between self-awareness and self-criticism is key to healthy resilience.

Self-critical talk can amplify the negative. It can diminish self-worth, making clinicians less likely to try new things in the future or seek opportunities for further learning. A pattern of dwelling on negative experiences – for example, an error made 20 years ago – can outweigh in the mind's eye multiple positive experiences since then – such as a grateful patient or a challenging but correct diagnosis. The concept of *negativity bias* is explored further in Chapter 3.

Conversely, self-awareness allows us to reflect on events from a more objective standpoint, focusing on what happened and how clinicians can learn and move on from these situations. This can build confidence and allow us to flourish professionally. In their systematic review, Mann *et al.* (2009) discuss the importance of reflective practice for building self-awareness as a tool to self-monitor and self-regulate our practice. Regular reflection on practice, particularly in partnership with skilled mentoring, promotes active learning and maintains competence. We develop as a reflective

---

ABC of Clinical Resilience, First Edition. Edited by Anna Frain, Sue Murphy, and John Frain.
© 2021 John Wiley & Sons Ltd. Published 2021 by John Wiley & Sons Ltd.

Box 4.1 **Physician Heal Thyself (??).**

These are the duties of a physician: first … to heal his mind and to give assistance to himself before giving it to anyone (else).

– Epitaph of an Athenian doctor, AD 2

The secret of the care of the patient is caring for oneself while caring for the patient.

– Rephrased by Lucy Candib 1995

Box 4.2 **The imposter syndrome.**

The *imposter syndrome* was a term first used by psychologists Suzanna Imes and Pauline Rose Clarence in the 1970s. It is not a recognised DSM-5 (Diagnostic and Statistical Manual of Mental Disorders) directive, but is common. It is suggested that 70% of people will experience it once in their life. It describes feelings of believing you are not as good as others perceive you to be and that you will be 'found out'.

Characteristics include:
- Self- doubt
- An inability to realistically assess your competence and skills
- Attributing your success to external factors
- Berating your performance
- Fear that you will not live up to expectations
- Overachieving
- Sabotaging your own success
- Setting very challenging goals and feeling disappointed when you fall short.

Source: Based on *What Is Imposter Syndrome?* by Arlin Cuncic, May 01, 2020. https://www.verywellmind.com/ (accessed 21.03.2021).

Table 4.1 Self-criticism versus self-awareness.

Event	Self-critical	Self-aware
Rejected for a job application	'I knew I was not good enough. I should never have applied. This is humiliating. Everyone else must be so much better than I am'.	'I'm disappointed, but it is okay. I understand not everyone gets their job choice. I will keep going. This is not a reflection on my self-worth. I can reflect on why I was rejected and use this to improve next time'.
Multiple unsuccessful attempts at performing a practical task	'I am terrible at this. I will never progress. Everyone else can do this easily. This is so shameful. Maybe I am not cut out for this career'.	'What am I missing? Where am I going wrong? Who can give me pointers? How can I get more practice to make this easier for me? I will get there'.
Made a mistake at work	'My bosses/the team are going to realise I'm not up to the task. They will find out I have never been good enough. My career is going to be ruined'.	'I made a human error. What did I learn? How can I change things so that this does not happen again? Can I help my colleagues not to make the same mistake as I did, and, if so, how? This mistake does not define me or my career'.

Box 4.3 **The reflective practitioner. How professionals think in action.**

Reflection in action (at the time the event is happening)	The experience itself Thinking about it during the event Deciding how to act at the time Acting immediately
Reflection on action (after the event)	Reflecting on something which has happened Thinking about what you might do differently if it happened again New information gained and/or theoretical perspectives from study that inform the reflector's experience are used to process feelings and actions

Source: Schon (1983). © 1984, Basic Books.

---

practitioner through appraisal and revalidation. Portfolios are a common mechanism used to help reflect on progress and make sense of experiences. Internal processes of reflection are also important. Schon's cycle of reflection, Box 4.3, encourages us to reflect in–and on–practice.

In his book titled *The Talent Code*, Daniel Coyle examines the psychology of people excelling in various fields, including music or sports (Coyle, 2009). He recommends 'operating at the edges of your ability', a phrase used to describe making mistakes to allow for the practice of error correction, to the point of being able to perform a task practically on autopilot. We learn through our unintentional mistakes. Healthcare advances often occur by learning from mistakes. BBC's 1987 TV series titled 'The Courage to Fail' recognised the development of many modern surgical techniques as resulting from this learning. Reflection allows us to identify our weaknesses and enables us to focus on our training and practice.

Tod *et al.* (2011) examined the effects of self-talk on performance in sport. They found that, in order to be beneficial and improve performance, self-talk should be positive, instructional and motivational. By using positive self-talk at work, we can improve the performance of practical tasks under pressure, just as sportspeople do on the field. Todd suggests that self-talk benefits cognition and movement skills, which could be likened to practical clinical skills and procedure competencies in the healthcare realm.

Self-awareness allows our outlook to remain balanced. A practical and simple way of starting this is to make an effort daily to let go of the difficulties and remember the positives as we leave work (Figure 4.1).

Schwartz rounds (see Chapter 7) have developed in primary and secondary care, initially in the USA. These allow shared reflections with colleagues and focusing on feelings and reactions to a situation rather than how it developed. These types of strategies are invaluable at challenging times such as during the Covid-19 pandemic.

Things to do as you leave work.

As part of self-care it is important to leave our work behind at the end of each day or each shift. Also we should try to concentrate on the positive and not the negative aspects of our work.

These are some suggestions to help us achieve this.

At the end of each shift;

- Take a moment to reflect on the day.
- Be proud of your work and the care you have given.
- Remember one difficult thing which has happened and let it go.
- Think about three positive things that have happened, however small. A patient saying thank you, a smile from a colleague or a diagnosis well made.
- Check on your colleagues and make sure they are OK.
- Are you OK? If not do you need to talk to someone or get some help?
- Make sure you go home to relax and leave your work behind you.

Adapted from a poster 'Going Home Checklist', Salford Care Organisation, Northern Care Alliance and Practitioner Health Programme presentation.

Figure 4.1 Self-care checklist Source: Designed by Doncaster and Bassetlaw Teaching Hospitals.

Resilience through the career cycle

The *threshold theory* (Land *et al.*, 2016) describes moving through the different stages of life and the resulting challenges as a series of transitions, leaving the familiar behind whilst progressing into strange and new territories. Understanding this as a normal process helps manage inherent anxieties, enabling satisfaction and growth. Moving through the following stages of a clinical career are examples of transitions:

- The healthcare student
- The first five years of qualification
- The established clinician
- The last five years

The healthcare student

Forming positive habits during student years (e.g., work–life balance, healthy eating, good sleep patterns) can serve as an excellent foundation for resilience throughout the career span (see Chapter 5). In his book titled *Why We Sleep*, Matthew Walker (2017) describes how even one night of impaired sleep can disrupt a student's ability to absorb new information and retain it in the short and long term. In addition, lack of sleep can lead to disrupted moods and altered eating habits – for example, making lower-quality food choices such as high-calorie sugary snacks more likely. Walker argues that planning ahead and ensuring we give ourselves adequate 'sleep opportunity' is an absolute essential for a healthy life.

Building restorative habits and a balance between the demands of studies and personal needs increases the likelihood of remaining resilient and coping better with potential burnout. In his hierarchy of needs, Maslow describes basic requirements which must be met in order for us to achieve our full potential (see Chapter 3, Figure 3.3). With the demands of training, even the most basic physiological needs may be unmet – for example, whilst studying

for an exam, missing meals can result in poor results, or scheduling restorative activities may be ignored. Activities such as scheduling a run or relaxing with friends can be invaluable. Students and professionals alike will perform much better, be more resilient and are more likely to deal with complex problems once their basic needs are met.

Avoiding negative coping strategies

Statistics paint a worrying picture of negative coping strategies for clinicians, including higher-than-average dependency on drugs and alcohol. If we adopt negative coping strategies clinical performance, patient care and clinician confidence are adversely affected which can lead to increased mental health problems. Table 4.2 outlines some positive and negative coping strategies.

Table 4.2 Summary of positive and negative coping strategies throughout a career.

	Positive coping strategies to develop	Negative coping strategies to avoid
Health professional student	Restorative behaviours Develop positive habits Study groups Peer support Plan and prepare Learn good study techniques	Poor sleep patterns Competitiveness
First five years	Ask for help Be aware of your limits Work as a team Use a reflective portfolio Communicate with clinical and educational supervisors	Leaving everything to the last minute
Experienced clinician	Find a mentor Build respect Network Be prepared to learn Pace yourself Learn to say 'no' Look after your well-being Develop your special interest	
Last five years	Plan ahead Recognise health issues. Work with your organisation Succession planning Financial planning Gradual reduction in workload/ responsibilities Develop post-retirement opportunities Consider teaching/ mentoring	Staying too long Avoiding early retirement if your mental or physical health is at stake.

Box 4.4 **Balint groups.**

Balint groups were started in the 1950s in the UK based on the work of the psychoanalyst Michael Balint. They provide an effective, safe, confidential and supportive setting for clinicians to reflect on their practice. Different professionals meet in groups of 6 to 10 for up 90 minutes to discuss cases with the help one or two facilitators. They try to explore the emotional content of the doctor–patient relationship, attempting to improve the understanding.

Michael Roberts describes the discussions in his group where he has met for 20 years, that they range from: *'the 'difficult' patient, making errors, work and home life balance, personal crises and illnesses, office challenges, medical learners, the 'system', joys of practice and the uniqueness of our relationships with our patients'.*

Source: Based on Roberts (2012).

Box 4.5 **Collaboration.**

Medical school can often have a competitive atmosphere, which can feel challenging at best, draining and doubt-inducing at worst. Choosing to work and study with your fellow students can turn this competition into collaboration. Splitting learning objectives into topics for each group member to research and then regrouping and teaching each other can be helpful. Using strategies that mimic exams, such as question banks to test each other, is proven to be far more effective than simply reading and re-reading course material as a revision method.

Source: Based on Roediger and Butler (2010).

Systemic causes of stress leading to poor coping strategies are discussed in later chapters (Chapters 6, 7 and 8). However, as reflective and self-aware practitioners, we can try to recognise when we are not coping. There are many simple factors that we can look at in order to manage stress:

- Sleep
- Diet
- Exercise
- Taking allocated annual leave
- Maintaining social networks
- Engaging in reflective practice (e.g., a Balint group – see Box 4.4)
- Mentoring.

Modern clinical practice requires teamwork, and training is the opportunity to learn do this well. Fellow trainees become life-long colleagues upon whom we will need to depend for support and who will also require our help (see Box 4.5). Ultra-competitiveness during training and beyond inhibits teamwork and, ultimately, patient safety.

The first five years of qualification

However well-prepared graduates are, entering the workplace as a newly qualified clinician can be daunting (see Box 4.6).

Box 4.6 **The foundation doctor.**

I had been told that the first year as a doctor can be the most challenging of the career. However, as a graduate student who had worked in healthcare for several years prior to medical training, I naively thought it would be a straightforward transition. In reality, I struggled with the workload, the hours and, most of all, my own confidence. In medical school, we are taught through OSCEs to appear confident even when we are not sure of ourselves. I think this led me to think that I was somehow a failure if I did not appear confident at work and needed help. In reality, as soon as I learnt that the burden of looking after patients did not solely fall on my shoulders, and that asking for help when you are struggling is one of the most important requirements of any healthcare worker, things started to improve. Instead of viewing myself as someone who had to prove myself, I started to realise that I was the most junior person on the team and that it was okay – even expected – that I would not know all the answers and would not be able to solve all the problems by myself. Having the confidence to be aware of the limits of our abilities and to speak up when we need help creates a much safer environment for patients.

– Foundation doctor

In the UK, newly qualified doctors have an educational supervisor who is involved in supporting their training. The doctor in training engages with an ePortfolio and their Educational Supervisor carries out regular reports on the progress of the trainee. Clinical supervisors also observe and assess progress. Mentoring and a peer support network can be invaluable. For nurses transitioning from student to registered nurse, there is recognition that settling into their new roles and responsibilities can be a difficult time. A case study (Whitehead *et al.*, 2016) demonstrates preceptorship as a process of supporting this transition.

Work–life balance

Achieving the appropriate work–life balance while working in clinical care can be extremely challenging. This is explored further in Chapter 2. There can be a tendency in clinicians for the 'unconscious motivation to heal to be channelled into a relentless drive to work' (Ballatt *et al.*, 2020). This can result in an unhealthy work–life balance, with self-care not always appropriately prioritised. The wellness wheel is one way of reflecting on the balance in our lives between life, work and external factors, and there is one example in Figure 4.2.

As our career and personal lives change, so the balance will vary. For example, having a young family or a parent to care for can result in the need to change our work–life balance. Box 4.7 shows one example of using reflection to improve work–life balance.

Caroline Elton (2018) explains that work–life balance is often a factor which guides clinicians in their choice of speciality.

'Newly qualified doctors today are less willing to devote their entire lives to their patients, at the expense of their own families, than their predecessors were. The issue of work–life balance has a more significant impact on the specialities doctors choose to follow than it did in the past'.

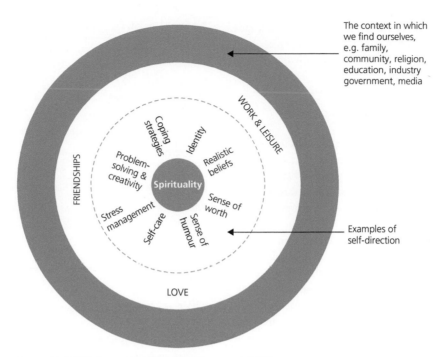

The context in which we find ourselves, e.g. family, community, religion, education, industry government, media

Examples of self-direction

Figure 4.2 Wheel of wellness, Cooper N. (2020). Source: Modified from Myers *et al.* (1998).

Box 4.7 **Vignette (positive coping strategy).**

One year at Christmas, my Mum bought myself and all of my siblings a beautiful notebook. She told us it was our 'Happy Book', and that we should write in anything that had happened that day that made us smile. It took me a while to get into it, but now I regularly write in anything that has made me happy – compliments I received, things that made me laugh out loud, etc. It only takes me two minutes to write, but it has had a more profound effect on my mental well-being than I ever thought something so simple could. I now spend my days looking for good things I can write in my book. I notice more positivity in each day, and I really take it in and experience the moment. I suppose it is a form of mindfulness. I relive those positive moments when I write them down, and then again when I reread the book when I need a little pick-me-up. I think everyone should have a Happy Book in their life. Thank you, Mum!

She quotes the Director of Medical Education at the Association of American Medical colleges:

> *The millennials seem to be more inclined than previous generations of physicians to trade some of their income for more control of their hours'.*

She also describes 'role reversal', where students can be indoctrinated to feel they are different from patients and can have great difficulty in being both a doctor and a patient at the same time. This can lead to clinicians delaying accessing help for both physical and psychological problems, resulting in worse outcomes.

The Covid-19 pandemic of 2020 has heightened recognition that clinicians and carers need a good work–life balance. Tools have been developed to assist clinicians – for example, the University of Nottingham toolkit (see the 'Further reading/resources' section).

The established clinician

You finally made it! Congratulations on your new role as a consultant, general practitioner, senior nurse or allied health professional. You are about to embark on an important transition in your working life. And, looking ahead, it might be useful to think about your career developing in three phases, each over a number of years – so pace yourself!

- Establishing yourself in the role
- Developing your special interest
- Becoming an expert

You (and your colleagues) have something valuable to offer at every stage of the career. As you find your feet, remember that you will get most respect by how you behave. A bad reputation can be quickly earned and difficult to shake off, while a good one comes with work but will endure.

You know a lot, but there is much to learn – and it is OK to ask for help. Seek out someone you trust for a safe place to offload. Focus on networking and learning how your organisation works.

This might be the first time you lead a team; you will achieve more by being a good listener. Your new responsibility will give you opportunities to inspire, challenge, teach, motivate and empower. Be generous – make sure everyone feels appreciated rather than taken for granted.

Make your own physical and mental well-being a priority. Be open to learning about strategies to help when times are tough, such as the art of saying 'no' when you are overwhelmed.

In some years, you too might be welcoming a new colleague. Remember how you felt, be explicit with the support you can offer and be generous with all that you have learned, now that you are considered to be wise.

When healthcare does not go as expected: The second victim

During a career in the health professions, there is likely to be a time when you or a colleague are involved in a complaint, claim, inquest or serious investigation. If this is something you have already experienced, how did it feel, what helped and what made things worse? Did the event lead to positive outcomes and quality improvements, or leave an indelible personal scar?

In 2000, Albert Wu coined the term 'second victim' and defined this as a healthcare provider involved in an unanticipated adverse patient event and/or medical error who is traumatised by the event.

The individual may initially experience a mixture of disorientation, detachment, agitation, anxiety, low mood, impaired judgment, confusion or amnesia. All these are recognised features of an acute stress reaction. Just to be able to acknowledge that this is an expected and very normal response may be helpful.

Negative thoughts may last from days to weeks and might involve reliving the event as well as feelings of shame, guilt, anger and self-doubt. Over time and with the right support, the feelings will subside, but there is a potential for recurrent re-traumatisation, especially where a process is long and drawn out such as litigation. Persistent thoughts lasting more than a month might be suggestive of post-traumatic stress disorder.

For individuals, needing support is entirely normal, and it might be helpful to talk to trusted colleagues, family and friends. Be aware of unhelpful behaviours such as repressing your emotions, defensive practices and avoidance of certain presentations. While the thought of talking with a patient or their family about an adverse event might be anxiety-provoking, this might be a positive step towards internal resolution.

If you have a colleague who is distressed, you maybe unsure how you might be able to help, but simply asking how they are managing, acknowledging that they have had a tough time and thanking them for sharing their thoughts with you may be therapeutic in itself. Be careful in sharing your own experiences or 'war stories'; while it may be helpful to hear that a trusted, experienced colleague has had their own experience of adverse events, your primary role is to be a good listener and not diminish a colleague's current difficulties by comparison. Avoid telling someone to 'get over it', and remember that the worse thing is to say is nothing at all.

For teams, departments and practices, support structures start with an acknowledgment that adverse events happen and can and will cause distress. Senior staff have a responsibility to ensure that the processes for investigation or case review are understood and normalised, and that they act as role models in their own approach to enable colleagues to feel safe to explore the events and to be constructive and creative in learning from opportunities.

The last five years

The last five years will have its' own challenges – see Table 4.3.

Table 4.3 The last five years.

Have I achieved a good enough work–life balance to continue to work safely and healthily?

Do I feel burnt out? I might retire too soon, waste wisdom and experience and regret my decision.

Do I wish to change the emphasis in my roles – perhaps do less clinical work and more academic/teaching commitment?

Am I recruiting my successor ensuring stability for my dental/physiotherapy/medical practice when I retire?

Do I have specific health issues which need to be considered?

What is the best way to reduce workload whilst sharing knowledge and experience with younger colleagues?

For a female clinician, am I tackling added complications such as the glass ceiling or menopause?

A Canadian study of surgeons summarises:

'Most surgeons wish to establish retirement plans that allow for the gradual reduction of surgical patient care and the creation of job opportunities for younger colleagues balanced by a continued contribution to the profession'.

Sharing clinical experience with younger colleagues can be an invaluable part of mentoring them. Small changes, reduced sessions and responsibilities passed to younger team members could prolong a career.

A Scandinavian study published in 2015 found that emotional exhaustion associated with older age, fear of litigation and feelings of isolation at work can be common in general practice. Statistics about age of death depending on age of retirement are sobering.

Caroline Elton describes how hard it can be for doctors to leave their profession when it clearly does not suit them and how it may actually cause them great harm. This is echoed in a Canadian study titled 'Doctors who retire early often met with scorn.' It is sometimes necessary for doctors to leave the profession early. They need to do what is best for them, their families as well as for their patients.

Finding the most positive way to spend your last five years could help prevent early retirement. Benefits can include improved patient care, increased personal satisfaction and an ability to encourage and support younger professionals.

Some useful tips on how individuals and organisations can work to support clinicians in their last five years are set out in Table 4.4.

Conclusions

Self-care is part of being a good clinician, yet we can fail to prioritise this. Understanding the varying pressures at different stages of our careers and developing our own toolbox to look after ourselves can result in a longer and more satisfying career. Accepting that we may all need help and support, and that things may go wrong, and being open and prepared to help others will help create a healthy and supportive working environment.

Table 4.4 A systematic review of physician retirement planning.

Things that result in early retirement	Excessive workload	Poor health	Low job satisfaction.		
Things that result in planned/delayed retirement	Strong work identity	Career satisfaction	Institutional flexibility	Financial obligations	
Strategies supporting continuing practice	Flexible work hours	Minimal work barriers	Enhancing work satisfaction	Financial planning	Physician health
Future research and strategies	Impact of flexible physician work hours	Gradual reduction in responsibilities	Resources for financial planning		
Creation of meaningful activity after retirement	Retirement resources toolkits	Education sessions	Financial planning through career	Post-retirement opportunities	Peer review, teaching, mentoring

A review of 65 international studies looking at the average age of retirement (60–69), reasons for early and late retirement and value of planning personally and as an institution. They summarise: *Preparation for a retirement that is tailored to physicians' career stages and specific age can avoid the complications that arise when a physician's career trajectory does not correspond to his or her expectations or what is in the best interests of the medical practice plan.*
Source: Based on Silver *et al.* (2016).

Further reading/resources

Ballatt, J., Campling, P. and Maloney, C. (2020) *Intelligent Kindness. Rehabilitating the Welfare State*. Cambridge University Press, Cambridge, UK.

Coyle, D. (2009) *The Talent Code*. Arrow Books, Bantum, New York.

Elton, C. (2018) *Also Human: The Inner Lives of Doctors*. Windmill Books, UK.

GP-S. Available at: https:/www.gp-s.org.

Land, R., Meyer, J.H.F. and Flanagan, M.T. (2016) *Threshold Concepts in Practice*. Sense Publishers, Rotterday, Taipei & Boston.

Mann, K. *et al.* (2009) Reflection and reflective practice in health professions education: a systematic review. *Advances in Health Sciences Education: Theory and Practice*, **14** (4), 595–621. PMID:18034364

Myers, J. E. (1998). *The Wellness Evaluation of Lifestyle Manual*. Mindgarden, Palo Alto, CA.

NHS Practitioner Help Programme. Available at: www.php.nhs.uk.

Phillips, A. and Taylor, B. (2010) *On Kindness*. Penguin, London.

Roberts, M. (2012) Balint groups: A tool for personal and professional resilience. *Canada Family Physician*, **58** (3), 245.

Roediger, H. and Butler, A. (2011) The critical role of retrieval practice in long-term retention. *Trends in Cognitive Sciences*, **15** (1), 20–27.

Hewitt, S. and Kennedy, U. (2020) *EM-POWER: A Wellness Compendium for EM*. Royal College of Emergency Medicine, London.

Schon, D. (1983) *The Reflective Practitioner. How Professionals Think in Action*. Basic Books, London.

Silver, M.P., Hamilton, A.D., Biswas, A. and Warrick, N.I. (2016) A systematic review of physician retirement planning. *Human Resources for Health*, **14** (1), 67. DOI: 10.1186/s12960-016-0166-z. PMID: 27846852; PMCID: PMC5109800.

Tod, D., Hardy, J. and Oliver, E. (2011) Effects of self-talk: a systematic review. *Journal of Sport and Exercise Psychology*, **33** (5), 666–687.

Walker, M. (2017) *Why We Sleep*. Penguin, UK.

Website for University of Nottingham Toolkit. Developed During the Covid Crisis. Available at: https://www.nottingham.ac.uk/toolkits/play-22794

Whitehead, B., Owen, P., Henshaw, L. *et al.* (2016) Supporting newly qualified nurse transition: a case study in a UK hospital. *Nurse Education Today*, **36**, 58–63.

Wu, A.W. (2000) The doctor who makes the mistake needs help too. *BMJ*, **320**, 726.

CHAPTER 5

The Physiology of Resilience and Well-being

Carla Stanton

Functional Medicine Doctor, Hertfordshire, UK

OVERVIEW

- Under sustained stress, autonomic, hormonal and cortical functions are compromised.
- Among the most sensitive markers of stress and well-being are heart rate variability and heart coherence.
- Combining biofeedback technology with scientifically validated self-regulation techniques can reduce the negative physiological impact of stress in real-time.
- Regular application of self-regulation techniques can entrain a new physiological baseline, promoting long-term resilience and well-being.
- Integrating techniques which promote physiological resilience into undergraduate and postgraduate training could reduce the incidence of burnout and improve patient outcomes.

Introduction

From restless nights before exams to fatigue following tough on-calls, all of us have experienced the detrimental physiological effects of stress at one time or another.

While the thousands of neurochemicals released during stress response help us in the short-term (e.g., by jumping into action when the crash bleep sounds or when pulling an 'all-nighter' to meet a deadline), chronic stress leads to a compromise in autonomic, hormonal and cortical functions.

In general, the stress and relaxation response are involuntarily regulated. However, several emerging fields of study, including psychoneuroendocrinology, neurocardiology and biofeedback technologies, are deepening our understanding of these responses, and demonstrating how it is possible to consciously influence them, reducing the detrimental impact of stress, to promote physiological resilience and well-being.

In this chapter, you will learn about the key physiological distinctions between stress and well-being. Techniques which entrain physiological baselines of resilience will also be discussed to better navigate these challenging times in healthcare.

The physiology of stress and well-being

The autonomic nervous system (ANS) regulates the majority of unconscious physiological processes essential to sustain life. This is possible through two opposing mechanisms: the stress response (via the sympathetic nervous system), and the relaxation response (through the parasympathetic nervous system).

The stress response ('fight or flight') is our innate ability to adapt to an environmental challenge in order to survive in the short term. The relaxation response – or 'rest and digest'/'feed and breed' – promotes a longer-term mechanism, restoring homeostasis once the threat has subsided.

The sympathetic system, when activated (neurochemically by noradrenaline, or NA), optimises the body's capacity to meet a physical challenge (i.e., run or fight) by increasing the heart rate, shutting off digestion, diverting more blood to muscle tissues, etc. The parasympathetic system, when stimulated (primarily via the vagus nerve by acetylcholine, or ACh), works to restore balance, thus promoting maintenance, growth and repair – and does this by slowing down the heart rate and diverting blood back to the central viscera (Figure 5.1).

The stress response is facilitated hormonally by the hypothalamic–pituitary–adrenal (HPA) axis (see Figure 5.2). Under stress, the hypothalamus releases corticotropin-releasing hormone (CRH), which stimulates the anterior pituitary gland to produce adrenocorticotropic hormone (ACTH). This signals the adrenal cortex to release catabolic glucocorticoids (mainly cortisol). When stress subsides, cortisol production is reduced, and anabolic hormones that are crucial for repair, such as dehydroepiandrosterone (DHEA) and oxytocin, are upregulated.

Through the continual counterbalancing influences of both the ANS and the HPA axis, our physiology rapidly adapts to stress, and quickly returns to well-being following a challenge.

From an anthropological perspective, this mechanism is well adapted for the significant and infrequent stress faced by human beings 200,000 years ago (such as chasing prey or fighting in conflict). These days, however, modern life has created a completely different landscape of stress, profoundly influencing this highly sophisticated system.

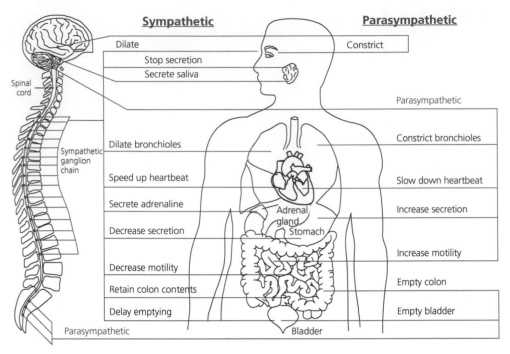

Figure 5.1 How the Autonomic Nervous System (ANS) innervates and influences the major organs of the body. Source: McCraty (2015). © 2020, HeartMath Institute.

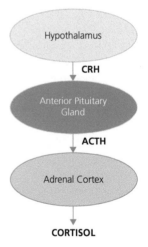

Figure 5.2 Activation of the hypothalamic–pituitary–adrenal (HPA) axis under stress.

The physiological impact of stress today

In today's society, stress is no longer an infrequent significant event, but a succession of repetitious minor stressors. For healthcare professionals, the challenges of increasing medical complexity and high patient turnover can mean that the stress response is activated throughout the day.

The physiological impact of stress can also be amplified by our neocortex, such that our own negative thoughts can significantly heighten real-world challenges. When we recall an unpleasant memory from our past (e.g., a traumatic patient event) or imagine a stressful event in our future (e.g., an upcoming set of on-calls with minimal staffing), we stimulate the stress response by thought alone. A clinical example of this is given in Box 5.1.

Box 5.1 **How thoughts influence our physiology: a familiar scenario.**

John, a fit and healthy 45-year-old plumber, attended a routine check-up with his GP and was found to have a high blood pressure of 165/89 mmHg and a heart rate of 88 bpm. As John's medical history and examination did not support any reason for these findings (John was also not feeling anxious, nor had he rushed to his appointment), John's GP arranged ambulatory home blood pressure monitoring for two weeks. All the home readings were normal (average 132/80 mmHg, heart rate 72 bpm). Following further discussions, John's GP concluded that he was exhibiting 'white coat syndrome'. In John's case, the 'pressure' of having his blood pressure taken had triggered a very mild stress response, increasing his heart rate and blood pressure. This was so minor that John did not 'feel stressed', but nonetheless his response was significant enough to cause a shift in his usual physiology, raising his heart rate and blood pressure above his normal physiological baseline. Reassured, they agreed on intermittent home blood pressure monitoring.

Whenever we remember a negative event from our past or anticipate a future one, whether real or imagined, helpful or unhelpful, the activation of the ANS and HPA axis triggers physiological effects downstream. In the short term, the effects are small, and the impact is minimal. However, over time, frequent thoughts of regret about the past, or worry about the future, result in a subtle but frequent low-stress state.

Over the course of months, chronically induced low-level stress shifts physiological baselines, such that high cortisol and higher levels of sympathetic activity can become 'the norm'. This is termed *high allostatic load*, the incapacity to return to a physiological baseline of well-being following stress, and this is what ultimately leads to physiological dysfunction.

'Challenge stress' versus 'threat stress'

To understand how this relates in practice, Figure 5.3 outlines the relationship between challenge and performance, and the corresponding physiological states.

When faced with a challenge (e.g., starting a new ward placement), the body expends energy. A small degree of sympathetic activation enables the body to move from point A of normal parasympathetic activity towards point B of 'healthy pressure'. Here, the parasympathetic and sympathetic activities become equally balanced. In the example of starting a new placement, this could be 'induction week', and is a point at which we learn very efficiently.

As the challenge continues – for example, we start working solo on the wards – we 'up the ante' by entering a sympathetically driven state to reach optimal performance at point C. You may have experienced this flow state for yourself when thriving in a new job role, achieving the perfect balance of challenge and performance – for example, feeling comfortable and competent performing certain clinical procedures required of your role. This physiological state is what makes a demanding job in healthcare feel incredibly satisfying, and is known as 'challenge stress'.

If the challenge continues (e.g., there is now an unfilled vacancy in your team, and you have to cover the extra workload), we reach a point where we perceive a shift at D. Here, the challenge is no longer a satisfying one – now it is overwhelming. If we do not restore the body back to balance (by moving back towards point A), the body continues to point E – threat stress. This does not initially compromise health (indeed, we can still perform quite well), but the important distinction is that we now perceive an emotional shift; what was once a pleasurable challenge now feels unpleasant and intimidating. This emotional shift can drive the chronic activation of the HPA axis, resulting in higher cortisol and lower DHEA levels. Here, at point E, sympathetic overdrive and high cortisol can

create symptoms such as hyper-vigilance, irritability, poor focus, anxiety and frustration.

Continual challenge eventually leads to a dysregulation of the ANS (point F) and a further compromise in DHEA and oxytocin. This depleted state (energetically via ANS and hormonally via HPA axis) is frequently termed 'burnout' (point G), which is a complex system of endocrine and immunological phenomena resulting in physical, mental and/or emotional exhaustion following periods of sustained high stress (De Vente *et al.*, 2015).

Measuring stress and well-being: heart rate variability and coherence

One of the most sensitive markers of ANS function is heart rate variability (HRV). Distinct from heart rate, HRV measures the variation in time intervals between adjacent heartbeats and is a real-time indicator of autonomic activity and capacity (Figure 5.4).

The role of HRV was noted as far back as 1965, when it was observed that foetal distress was preceded by a reduction in HRV before a change in heart rate (Hon *et al.*, 1965). HRV is now a well-established biomarker for health, reducing by an average of 3–5% per year. An abnormally low HRV relative to one's age is a strong and independent predictor of future health problems, including all-cause mortality (Tuomainen *et al.*, 2005). To date, there have been several cross-sectional studies demonstrating lower levels of HRV in conditions such as depression and anxiety, as well as behaviours such as rumination and self-criticism. Conversely, studies indicate a positive correlation between well-being and HRV, with renewing practices such as practicing compassion increasing HRV (Kirby *et al.*, 2017).

The regularity of the rhythm is also important and is known as *coherence*. More uniform heart rhythm cycles, the greater the coherence, reflecting an optimal balance of sympathetic and para-sympathetic outflow and to the person's DHEA: cortisol levels (McCraty, 2015). (Figure 5.5)

Greater coherence is associated with improved emotional well-being, DHEA levels and positive health effects (McCraty, 2015). In contrast, incoherent patterns are correlated with poorer out-

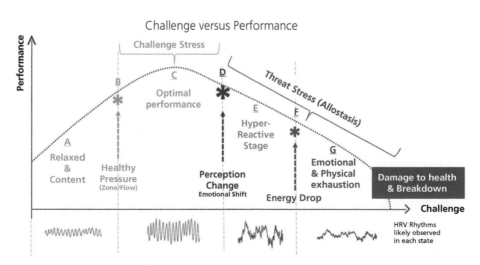

Figure 5.3 The relationship between challenge and performance. Source: Yerkes and Dodson (1908) and McCraty (2015). © 2020, HeartMath Institute.

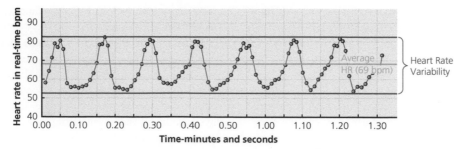

Figure 5.4 The relationship between heart rate (HR) and heart rate variability (HRV). Source: Screenshot with permission from HeartMath emWave Software.

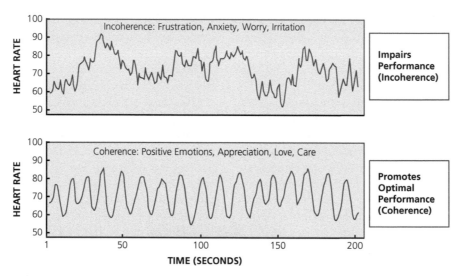

Figure 5.5 Incoherent versus coherence heart rhythms. Source: McCraty (2015). © 2020, HeartMath Institute.

comes, and have been observed alongside HRV dysregulation in physiologically demanding roles such as nurses working night shifts (Burch *et al.*, 2019).

Cortical inhibition and facilitation

Heart rhythms also influence cortical function (via the vagus nerve, a key component of the parasympathetic nervous system). For the healthcare worker, this means that threat stress can result in impaired focus, clinical reasoning and communication, with potential impact on patient safety. This is because the majority of the vagus nerve (80%) is composed of afferent fibres, which means that most of the information between the heart and the brain is ascending. This means that the rhythms produced by the heart profoundly influence the activity of the amygdala in the midbrain, and therefore the information that is relayed to the neocortex.

Incoherent heart rhythms created by threat stress activate the amygdala to induce behavioural, immunological and neuroendocrine responses favouring survival. Under threat stress, the incoherent rhythm induces 'cortical inhibition' of perceptual, cognitive and emotional processes (Kirby *et al.*, 2017). This explains the 'brain freeze' phenomenon – when acute stress (e.g., being affronted by an angry relative) inhibits one's capacity to think logically and communicate clearly (e.g., we say something we regret, or nothing at all) (Figure 5.6). This is incredibly pertinent for healthcare

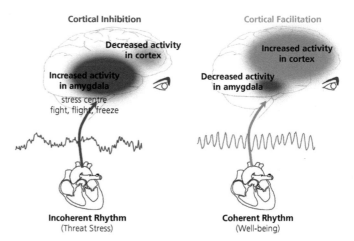

Figure 5.6 How heart rhythms influence cortical activity. Source: McCraty (2015). © 2020, HeartMath Institute.

workers, who work in challenging environments and need to consistently be able to communicate effectively and make safe clinical decisions. Fortunately, there are simple techniques which can be applied during threat stress that induce more coherent heart rhythm patterns, thereby promoting cortical facilitation. There is a strong argument for all healthcare professionals to develop this skill in order to mitigate the negative physiological impact of threat stress and promote patient safety.

Making a shift: influencing HRV and coherence

Thanks to the unique anatomy of the vagus nerve, it is possible to consciously influence HRV and coherence and induce positive physiological changes. The vagus nerve is the fastest acting and longest nerve of the body, with extensive visceral connections throughout, which means that techniques targeting the vagus nerve can induce rapid and widespread effects on the brain and body. This grants us the capacity to promote a physiological state of well-being when we begin to enter threat stress.

The therapeutic potential of vagus nerve stimulation devices is widely researched, while breathing practices which trigger the vagus nerve to induce a pattern change via respiratory sinus arrhythmia (thus instantaneously increasing HRV and coherence) are often underestimated.

Research demonstrates that resonant frequency breathing (RFB), which is deep and regular breathing (typically at six breaths/minute, or 0.1 Hz), is one of the most effective ways to induce coherence and increase HRV (Steffen *et al.*, 2017), promoting a physiology of well-being.

The physiology of emotion

Emotions play a crucial role in physiological function and heart rhythms. Building on the phases (A–G) described in the 'Challenge versus Performance' graphic, Figure 5.7 illustrates the physiological manifestations of renewing (broadly positive) and depleting (broadly negative) emotions (via the ANS and HPA axis).

Take a moment now to look at this grid, and ask yourself: are there any particular emotions or quadrants that represent your own lived experience day to day? Your emotions will inevitably depend largely on the challenges of your day – but, over time, repeated emotional states can entrain the ANS and HPA axis to certain physiological patterns or habits. Take a few moments to consider: 'What is your emotional landscape, and what information might this give you about your current physiological baseline?'

The demands of a career in healthcare (and life in general) will inevitably bring with it a rich tapestry of emotions, both renewing and depleting. However, we do have the capacity to reduce the amount of time we may spend in unhelpful and depleting emotional states. Research has shown that it is not the objective challenge alone, but our subjective perception of that challenge which seems to have the biggest impact in the switch from challenge to threat stress. A study on caregivers of chronically ill children investigated the influence of stress perception on telomere length. (Telomeres are the DNA–protein structures found at the ends of each chromosome. Every time a cell divides, telomeres gets shorter; thus, their length serves as a biological marker of age and well-being.) The study concluded that, despite equal objective stressors, caregivers who perceived their challenge as 'threat stress' had significant telomere shortening, while caregivers who perceived it as 'challenge stress' preserved much more telomere length (Epel *et al.*, 2004).

Physiological resilience is thus the capacity to:

- Promptly perceive when we switch into depleting emotional states of threat stress (point D)
- Take appropriate action, by either reducing the challenge, or changing our perception of it

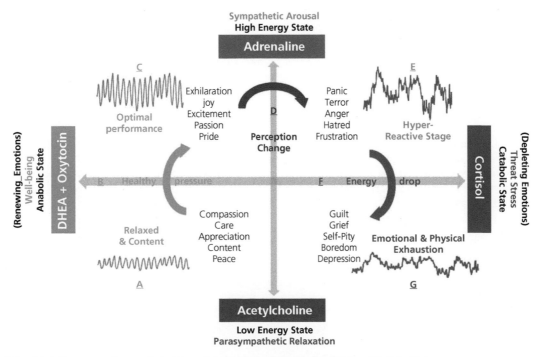

Figure 5.7 The relationship between emotions and physiology. Source: McCraty (2015). © 2020, HeartMath Institute.

Becoming aware of a perception change

Perceiving a switch from renewing to depleting emotions requires that we become familiar with our inner emotions and thoughts and observe how we express them through our actions and behaviours. The majority of the time, we are completely unaware of these traits, because the default mode network (often described as 'the voice in our head'), with its extensive connections throughout the brain, is created through unconscious habit. This means that the vast majority of our 60,000–70,000 thoughts a day (and their associated emotions) are both repetitious and unconscious. Fortunately, the neocortex affords us the ability to objectively observe our thoughts. We can begin to 'think about what we think about'; a process called *metacognition*. A practical application is indicated in Box 5.2.

Figure 5.8 demonstrates how each physiological state can relate to the thoughts of our inner world, and how we express them through our behaviours.

These diagrams illustrate how repeated and often unconscious patterns of recurrent emotions, thoughts and behaviours neurochemically influence our physiology, and can ultimately mould our personality over time. Metacognitive practices such as mindfulness and meditation grant insight into these unconscious habitual processes, thus enabling us to identify and change any unhelpful patterns by consciously selecting new thoughts, emotions and behaviours. Such self-regulation strategies have been shown to increase resilience and recovery from threat stress, as well as improve cardiac coherence (McCraty and Zayas, 2014).

> Box 5.2 **Practical application of metacognition on the night shift.**
>
> Christina, an ST2 GP trainee, is on her final shift of nights working as the only A&E doctor in a remote hospital. The week has been especially challenging, and she is aware of feeling progressively more irritable and impatient. At 4 am, she is called to see a young man with severe shoulder pain who has fallen while out drinking. She diagnoses a simple anterior shoulder dislocation and must coordinate safe relocation of the shoulder under sedation. In normal circumstances, she would feel confident to coordinate this with her nursing team, but she is practicing metacognition, and having observed her increasingly negative thoughts, behaviours and emotions throughout the past week, she is aware of the increased risk posed by her depleted physiological state. As such, she requests assistance from the on-call orthopaedic registrar, and the procedure is undertaken safely and successfully.

Making the shift back to well-being

Just as an athlete must train to perform on race day, healthcare professionals need to regularly practice self-regulation techniques to make safe and effective clinical decisions consistently under pressure.

By combining RFB with emotional self-regulation techniques and biofeedback technology, it is possible to create new physiological baselines within a relatively short period of time. Research shows that just five minutes of practice, three times a day, for as little as 28 days, can bring about positive changes in healthcare workers, PTSD victims and schoolchildren (Lemaire *et al.*, 2011, Ginsberg *et al.*, 2010, Bradley *et al.*, 2010; see Box 5.3).

A study by the US Department of Education demonstrated that these techniques can significantly reduce test anxiety, and improve test scores, HRV and coherence. Figure 5.9 shows the pre- and post-intervention measurements from two students who remained dedicated to self-regulation practices over four months (Bradley *et al.*, 2010). Box 5.4 shows an example case study.

Conclusion

With health service pressures set to rise over the next 20 years (GMC Annual Report, 2018), it is critical that we prioritise the physiological well-being of our clinical workforce by adopting scientifically validated strategies to better prepare for, adapt to and recover from the increasing challenges of working in clinical care.

Biofeedback research is providing promising data on the potential of simple self-regulation techniques to promote physiological well-being in time-pressured clinical care workers.

It is possible that, by combining biofeedback technology with scientifically validated self-regulation techniques, a healthcare professional could be taught how to recognise stress more quickly, apply a self-regulation technique in the moment and make more effective clinical decisions by reducing the detrimental physiological impact of stress.

Over time, such practices have the potential to improve the physiological flexibility of healthcare workers and reduce the incidence of burnout. Perhaps more significantly, a healthcare workforce skilled in self-regulation could make safe and effective clinical decisions more consistently, improving patient experience and safety.

Further research is needed into the application of such strategies, which have the potential to improve well-being, clinical competence and patient outcomes at every stage of clinical training and beyond.

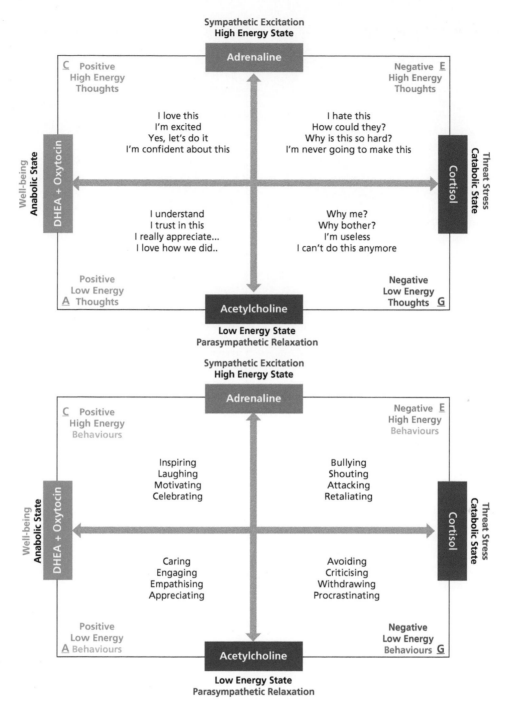

Figure 5.8 The physiological relationship between thoughts and behaviours. Source: McCraty (2015). © 2020, HeartMath Institute.

Box 5.3 **The Quick Coherence Technique for self-regulation.**

The Quick Coherence Technique (QCT) is a scientifically validated self-regulation technique developed by the HeartMath Institute. The technique can be performed with eyes open or closed, and is a simple, three-step process for inducing heart coherence in the moment. You should practice it for 1–5 minutes to obtain the physiological benefit. It is a helpful tool to prepare for a stressful event (e.g., a challenging consultation) or recover from a stressful experience (e.g., a trauma call).

Step 1. Focus your attention in the area of the heart. You can do this by gently placing your palm or two fingers over your heart area.
Step 2. Imagine your breath is flowing in and out of your heart or chest area, and breathe a little slower and deeper than usual. To achieve resonant frequency breathing, inhale for five seconds, and exhale for five seconds.
Step 3. Try to experience a regenerative feeling such as appreciation or care for someone or something in your life. You might call to mind someone you love, a pet, a special place or an accomplishment to help you feel a sense of calm or ease.

Source: McCraty (2015). © 2020, HeartMath Institute.

Box 5.4 **Case study: Successful application of self-regulation.**

The account that follows is real and demonstrates the power of applying self-regulation in high-stress situations akin to those experienced by healthcare professionals. The data is supplied with the subject's permission (her name has been changed).

Sarah, 36, is a development director of a leading UK civil engineering company. After experiencing work-related stress and reading a paper in which nurses at Bart's Hospital successfully reduced stress through biofeedback and self-regulation (Riley and Gibbs, 2014), Sarah practiced these techniques, and recorded her biofeedback for five minutes twice daily for 15 months.

Sarah was practicing self-regulation while checking her emails on a normal working day when she received a phone call from her boss informing her that a fatal collision had just taken place on her project site. Sarah must now talk to the police, as well as her employees and clients. A screenshot of this moment is captured in Figure 5.10.

This was a grave professional tragedy, but Sarah quickly realised she had entered threat stress, and performed the 'shift and reset' technique (focusing on her heart and performing four resonant frequency breaths). The HRV tracing indicates that this was successful in immediately inducing high coherence before she disconnected the device and dealt with the situation. This was a hugely challenging experience, but Sarah reports being able to compassionately communicate and effectively coordinate all the unpleasant tasks of that day.

Source: McCraty (2015). © 2020, HeartMath Institute.

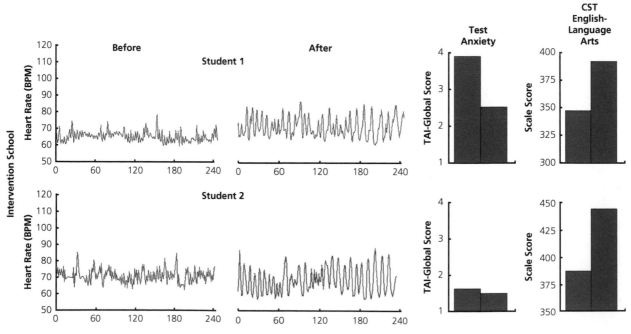

Figure 5.9 Improvements in students using regular self-regulation techniques. Source: McCraty (2015). © 2020, HeartMath Institute.

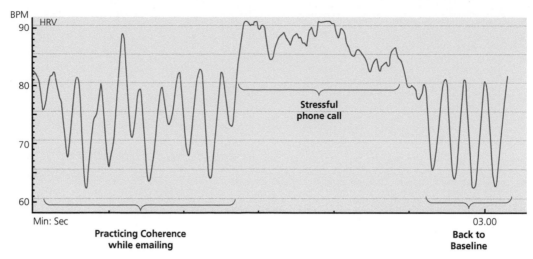

Figure 5.10 HRV tracing capturing Sarah's stressful moment. Source: Screenshot with permission from case-study subject and HeartMath emWave Software.

Further reading/resources

Boullier, M. and Blair, M. (2018) Adverse childhood experiences. *Paediatrics and Child Health*, **28** (3). 132–137.

Bradley, R.T., McCraty, R., Atkinson, M. *et al.* (2010) Emotion self-regulation, psychophysiological coherence, and test anxiety: results from an experiment using electrophysiological measures. *Applied Psychophysiology and Biofeedback*, **35** (4), 261–283.

Burch, J.B., Alexander, M., Balte, P. *et al.* (2019) Shift work and heart rate variability coherence: pilot study among nurses. *Applied Psychophysiology and Biofeedback*, **44**, 21–30.

De Vente, W., van Amsterdam, J.G.C., Olff, M. *et al.* (2015) Burnout is associated with reduced parasympathetic activity and reduced HPA axis responsiveness, predominantly in males. *BioMed Research International*, **2015** (2015): 431725.

Epel, E.S., Blackburn, E.H., Lin, J. *et al.* (2004) Accelerated telomere shortening in response to life stress. *Proceedings of the National Academy of Sciences*, **101** (49), 17312–17315.

Ginsberg, J.P., Berry, M.E. and Powell, D.A. (2010) Cardiac coherence and PTSD in combat veterans. *Alternative Therapies in Health and Medicine*, **16** (4), 52–60.

GMC Annual Report (2018). Available at: https://www.gmc-uk.org/-/media/documents/annual-report-2018-english_pdf-80413921.pdf.

Hon, E.H. and Lee, S.T. (1965) Electronic evaluations of the fetal heart rate patterns preceding fetal death: further observations. *American Journal of Obstetric Gynecology*, **87**, 814–826.

Kirby, J.N., Doty, J.R., Petrocchi, N., and Gilbert, P. (2017) The current and future role of heart rate variability for assessing and training compassion. *Frontiers in Public Health*, 08 March 2017.

Lemaire, J.B., Wallace, J.E., Lewin, A.M. *et al.* (2011) The effect of a biofeedback-based stress management tool on physician stress: a randomized controlled clinical trial. *Open Medicine*, **5** (4), 154–163.

McCraty, R. (2015) *Science of the Heart: Exploring the Role of the Heart in Human Performance, Volume* 2. HeartMath Institute, Boulderr Creek, California.

McCraty, R. and Zayas, M. (2014) Cardiac coherence, self-regulation, autonomic stability, and psychosocial well-being. *Frontiers in Psychology*, **5**, 1–13.

Riley, K. and Gibbs, D. (2014) Revitalizing care program in UK Healthcare: does it add up? *Global Advances in Health and Medicine*, **3** (Suppl 1), BPA10.

Steffen, P.R., Austin, T., DeBarros, A. and Brown, T. (2017) The impact of resonance frequency breathing on measures of heart rate variability, blood pressure, and mood. *Frontiers in Public Health*, **5**, 222.

Tuomainen, P., Peuhkurinen, K., Kettunen, R. and Rauramaa, R. (2005) Regular physical exercise, heart rate variability and turbulence in a 6-year randomized controlled trial in middle-aged men: the DNASCO study. *Life Sciences*, **77** (21), 2723–2734.

Yerkes, R. and Dodson, J. (1908) The relation of strength of stimulus to rapidity of habit-formation. *Journal of Comparative Neurology*, **18** (5), 459–482.

Websites

To learn more about the research behind heart coherence and its role in stress and emotional well-being, see: https://www.heartmath.org/resources/videos/scientific-foundation-of-the-heartmath-system

For a (downloadable) audio demonstration of a validated self-regulation technique from the HeartMath Institute, see: https://www.heartmath.org/resources/heartmath-tools/quick-coherence-technique-for-adults

UK resource for Schwartz Rounds, a group reflective practice forum which provides opportunities for staff from all disciplines to reflect on the emotional aspects of their work, see: https://www.pointofcarefoundation.org.uk/our-work/schwartz-rounds/

CHAPTER 6

Intelligent Kindness: A Systemic Perspective on Resilience

John Ballatt

The Openings Consultancy, Leicester, UK

OVERVIEW

- Resilience is not just down to the individual.
- The work always involves remaining open to, and managing, difficult feelings.
- Personality *and* the culture of the working environment influence how well such feelings are managed.
- Resilience, while involving 'self-care', is also promoted by self-awareness, reflective practice *and* the healthy collaboration between colleagues and the wider system.
- Kinship, and its expression through 'intelligent kindness' by clinicians in their relationships with each other and patients, promotes both effectiveness *and* staff well-being.
- Well-designed and managed systems of care, and healthy collaborative relationships, are crucial to the resilience of all.
- Leaders have a duty of care: they must cultivate a healthy 'kinship system', and work to minimise factors that undermine and distract from it.

Resilience and recovery – definitions and questions

The continued physical and emotional well-being of clinicians is vital to the effectiveness of all health services. This hardly revolutionary idea merits careful exploration in the context within which people work. Definitions of *resilience* refer to the ability to recover after a difficulty, to be tough – the capacity to 'spring back into shape' after being somehow twisted or crushed. There is the added sense that something will not be worn down by frequent use – all interesting concepts, and already raising issues. If work is continuously, day after day, characterised by 'difficulty', what does 'recovery' imply? What does 'toughness' do to humane, effective practice? What is involved in the 'elasticity' of springing back into shape – both in terms of the characteristics of the one who is crushed, and of the pressures and forces doing the crushing?

Reflection and self-care

While these definitions do refer to pressures that impact upon clinical staff, they can tend to place the focus too much on the individual. The question can become 'how can they look after themselves?' Of course, the ways individuals manage themselves is important. A range of valuable approaches can help, ranging from 'ordinary' things like good sleep, diet and exercise, to more specialist activities like mindfulness-based stress reduction (MBSR), compassionate mind training (CMT) or meditation. It is similarly very helpful for individuals to build the habit of reflective practice, with what Donald Schön called 'reflection-in-action' (carried out as one works) and 'reflection-on-action' (carried out in time and space set aside, and best helped by a skilled other) (Schön, 1983). There is a danger, however, that overemphasis on the individual can mean that we neglect addressing the factors that are doing the wearing down, causing the stress and undermining well-being.

The emotional costs of caring

Some aspects of the work are inescapable. At the centre of practice is the encounter between the clinician and the patient. *All* clinical work involves encounters with difficulty, on a spectrum from uncertainty – of diagnosis, prognosis, treatment and risk – through to feelings of revulsion, high anxiety and utter helplessness. All the time, staff, however fleetingly, are involved in relationships with fellow human beings, whose distress can make engagement difficult, confusing and painful. Clinicians bring their own vulnerabilities, insecurities, blind spots and conscious/unconscious motivations into their work, and not always helpfully. The circumstances of their day-to-day personal lives affect their mood, attention, energy and 'mental space' for others.

Of course, training and the journey into qualified practice gradually acclimatises the practitioner to such realities. Clinicians largely overcome natural human urges to gag, turn away, give up or even flee (see Box 6.1).

ABC of Clinical Resilience, First Edition. Edited by Anna Frain, Sue Murphy, and John Frain.
© 2021 John Wiley & Sons Ltd. Published 2021 by John Wiley & Sons Ltd.

Box 6.1 **Overcoming natural reactions.**

'As a medical student, I found myself fainting whilst simply observing painful procedures such as inserting a chest drain or doing a liver biopsy. I would start to feel hot, and, before I realised what was happening, I would be unconscious on the floor. It was quite a psychological slog to get over this. I had to stop looking the patient in the face and distance myself from their pain'.
　60-year-old doctor
　Personal communication

Box 6.2 **Experiences in the time of Covid-19.**

'It all happened so quickly. We seemed completely unprepared. I have never seen such ill patients and such horrible deaths – or indeed so many. There was always anxiety about PPE, and I had to make a fuss to find PPE in my size, which was rather embarrassing. At the end of my shift, I would scrub myself for ages in the shower, very anxious about what I would take home to my wife and vulnerable mother-in-law. And when I got home, I could not really talk about it all'.
　Junior doctor on ICU
　Quotation is an invention/anonymisation of communications

Box 6.3 **Demands and reality.**

'We are supposed to be a specialist psychotherapy service for people at the highest risk. Our waiting list is over a year, and I dare not tell you how many people are on it. There is constant pressure to take up 'new, effective treatment models' with the obvious agenda of speeding up 'throughput'. Though some of them might, indeed, be helpful, even cutting our number of sessions by half would not touch the waiting list in any convincing way. Anyway, our priority should be the patients. This is just so wearing and infuriating'.
　Senior NHS psychotherapist
　Anonymised and rephrased

Box 6.4 **Disrespect for practitioner experience and needs.**

1　The UK's health secretary's suggestion, in the midst of the worst of the Covid-19 pandemic, that staff overused PPE, instead of 'treating it as a precious resource', insulted and infuriated staff. Black and minority ethnic clinicians, already reported as less confident about asserting their needs for PPE, while also having a higher death rate, were even more reluctant. We will never know what the consequences in terms of fatalities were, but it takes little imagination to recognise the anxiety and preoccupation that will have infected practice.
2　A young nurse on an inpatient ward becomes aware that one of the patients has tested positive for Covid-19. She has a long-planned visit to her elderly grandparents at the weekend and asks if she can have a test. Her manager says 'no', and that it is not a priority. She is forced into a 70-mile roundtrip to get a test at a drive-in test centre.
　Public knowledge and personal communication from a relative

They 'get used to it'; learn to engage, to look closely, to refer to evidence and to think rationally; and develop a repertoire of interventions that will, or can, help. There is the danger that this journey leads to hardening, to less attentiveness to the experience of their patients. Notably, research suggests that, a few years into practice, medical and nursing staff appear to be less compassionate than when they began their training (see Sinclair, 1997). Is this, however, mainly to do with them as people, or as much, or more, to do with the effects of the system and culture in which they work?

In 2020, the public narrative that emerged surrounding the experience of healthcare staff as they initially faced Covid-19 highlights the importance of this question. Staff, individually and through their professional organisations, reported distress in the face of the suffering and anxiety of patients and their families. They have fears about their own, and their loved ones', vulnerability and weariness, coupled with the determination to carry on. But that story means little without context. These felt experiences happened in the face of real or predicted overwhelming demand, of fears generated by inadequate testing resources and shortages of clinical and personal protection equipment, beds and staff (see Box 6.2).

Though extreme in times of a pandemic, such factors, to varying extents, always influence the psychological well-being of individual staff, and of the teams and services within which they operate. The annual cycle of 'winter pressures', for example, often means an overwhelming surge of demand on staff. But they can simply be inherent in the system. GPs work, typically, in 10-minute appointments, within the context of often troubling delays for tests and specialist interventions. Psychotherapists, physiotherapists and speech therapists very frequently have to manage very high waiting lists – the result of a dangerous mismatch between staffing resources and need. Psychiatrists manage enormous caseloads, with inadequate community resources, shortages of acute beds and constant pressure to manage 'risk'. Hospital clinicians face the problems caused by a neglected social care sector that 'blocks' their beds, and by inadequately staffed, unstable nursing teams reliant on temporary staff. The optimism, energy, confidence and effectiveness of all healthcare staff are profoundly and chronically influenced by such experiences. At the very least, frustration, anger and anxiety are generated in many, with consequent effects on their own well-being and their capacity to practice (see Box 6.3).

If the nature of clinical practice and practical problems in the system are so influential, even more so is the psychological climate, the culture, of the organisations in which staff work. If minimisation, denial or blame by politicians, managers or colleagues are the perceived responses to their experience, staff are understandably mistrustful, angry or despairing (see Box 6.4).

If they experience consistent, open, honest and sympathetic acknowledgement – of the rigours of the clinical task itself, and of shortfalls and problems in the system – staff will be far less anxious, cynical or angry. If they experience respect and recognition of their personal worth and individuality, from managers, leaders and each other, clinicians will thrive far better. When staff feel that focused and committed attention is given, *as a priority*, to enabling their work, and addressing factors that undermine it, their sense of optimism, safety and trust will grow. These are core aspects of resilience.

Kinship

One way of looking at healthcare, and indeed all forms of care, is as a sophisticated expression of the evolutionary development and expression of *kinship*. Historically, many living things, and especially humans, developed and thrived by sharing risks, resources and opportunities. They achieved success by supporting each other as mutually dependent members of an ever-expanding circle of kinship. They did not just develop a sense of individual concern, of compassion, for the suffering 'other'. They expressed the reality that we are 'of a kind', that we depend on each other for our collective well-being. Such a perspective may be termed 'intelligent kindness' (Ballatt *et al.*, 2020). Compassion is, of course, vital, but can be readily reduced to the feelings of individuals, taking out of focus the challenge, and the responsibility, for the collective to nurture its members, as they nurture those they care for. Simply put, the well-being of patients *and* staff needs to be sustained by all, and for all, through *systematic* cultivation of the conditions within which they will thrive.

What does such an approach entail? It is helpful to begin by looking at the psychological aspects of the clinical task more closely.

A therapeutic alliance

At the heart of practice, whatever the technical aspects of care giving, lies the need to engage with the patient and their distress, to form an alliance with them to address their needs. The clinician, as a representative of the 'kinship' group, needs to engage sympathetically, 'kindlily', with their patient, to be attentive, to become attuned to their experience, needs and suffering. Such attention builds the trust that will promote openness, honesty and cooperation, which secure the alliance that will lead to the best possible outcomes we want (see Box 6.5).

For both clinician and patient, this process and these outcomes themselves strengthen the relationship and lay the foundations for further work. This can be seen as a virtuous circle (Figure 6.1). This way of looking at the work is supported by the lessons of *attachment theory* (Bowlby, 1969).

The benefits of compassion and kindness

It is important to recognise that such a way of working is vital to the technical aspects of the job. Diagnosis will be more accurate, treatment choices more likely to be optimal, cooperation in treatment improved and outcomes better. Seeing the work through this lens is as important for patient safety, effectiveness and efficiency as any care protocol or evidence-based treatment plan. Patients appreciate an encounter with 'kindness' or compassion; they feel better about the clinician and their treatment. But evidence suggests something more: treatment shaped by compassion is more effective. Wounds heal more quickly (Weinman *et al.*, 2008); over-users of A&E reduce their visits (Rendelmeir *et al.*, 1995); and psychological

> ### Box 6.5 **Trust and the therapeutic alliance.**
>
> 'The consultant who has been treating me does not fit my stereotype of the cold, distant, arrogant surgeon at all. After any examination, he always offers me a hand to help me get up from the examination table. I have found this small gesture of kindness very significant. It has helped me feel able to communicate with him in an open and honest way as a person, not just another ill patient.
>
> I have had complete trust in both the surgeon and the oncologist who have been treating me for cancer. Because of the trust I have in both of them, this has made the decision about what to do next very easy for me. I have not felt the need to examine statistics or trawl the Internet for information. I have felt confident in making my decision, given that my doctors, whilst being experts in their fields and having my best interests at heart, were also able and willing to empathise with me and with my situation'.
>
> Personal communication by a (now recovered) patient

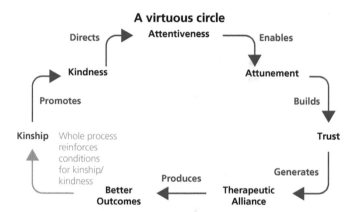

Figure 6.1 A Therapeutic Alliance. Source: Ballatt *et al.* (2020). © 2020, Cambridge University Press.

treatment (of any kind) works better if the patient experiences such a positive relationship (Bohart and Tallman, 1999).

Cultivating intelligent kindness

What, though, if we consider the implications for the staff? To engage in this way means that they need to have, day-after-day, the emotional and attitudinal readiness to bear others – their patients and each other – in mind. They need the imagination to understand both the other's experience, and how possible interventions might affect them. They need a sense of 'agency', of freedom to feel, think and act. An environment is required that fosters these qualities. This means that attention must be given to promoting and sustaining them – in the way staff experience each other in their teams, and in the way the organisations in which they work construct and influence their daily working lives. Staff thrive when they, themselves, experience the attention, understanding, support and cooperative fellowship illustrated in our virtuous circle.

What does a systemic approach to promoting resilience involve? In fact, there are two ways of looking at the system, which require equal, and joint, attention. It needs to be seen, at one and the same time, as a 'task and role' system, and as a 'kinship' or 'relational' system.

Healthcare services, whether delivering primary or acute care, are highly complex. They bring together a range of professional roles and functions, in teams and in wider systems, to meet needs that present themselves – sometimes predictably, very often not. They organise a range of managerial, administrative, logistical and governance processes. The match between the work and resources required and what is available is sometimes fine, sometimes dangerously uncertain. How well the roles, tasks and functions are designed, individually and as a system, has enormous influence on the confidence, goodwill, collaboration and effectiveness of staff in all roles, on their continued well-being. Great care is needed to keep the whole system in mind, despite factors that tend to undermine such a perspective. It is not helped by the often-fragmented nature of contracts for the many services that need to work together. The competitive nature of the 'market' can lead to over-promising, to reliance on unrealistic goals of 'efficiency', to self-interested 'parts', rather than cooperation as a whole system.

Figure 6.2 illustrates the various levels of the task and role system that require attention, at individual levels and as a whole system. The factors that can skew that work, and must be carefully managed to minimise that risk, are indicated in the outer circle.

However well designed and structured the system, how it is turned into reality by the human community at work makes the crucial difference. Much depends on the explicit and implicit *purpose* and *priorities* of people in various roles as they undertake tasks to make the system work. Determined effort needs to be made to encourage everyone, in every role, to make their primary focus collaboration with – and enabling – staff as they work with patients. Constant care is required to ensure that there is synergy between expectations, arrangements, targets, priorities and the lived experience of staff working 'at the frontline'. Morale and, indeed, well-being, are threatened if they experience the concerns of other parts of the system as distractions from, in contradiction to, skewing, or over-determining their focus on patients (see Box 6.6).

Factors that undermine the work

If the targets, for a care pathway or service, about numbers of patients treated, or 'throughput' achieved, are out of kilter with the needs being addressed, staffing levels or resources available, staff well-being will suffer. When one part of the system is designed with the expectation that other parts will play complementary roles, but they cannot, or will not, the consequent frustration and anxiety aroused can be toxic. When staff experience governance, performance management, health and safety or even CPD processes as intrusive, impractical, punitive or blind, this will chronically undermine their resilience. If the people responsible for such functions anxiously make meeting the expectations on *them* the priority, rather than enabling clinical practice, an unhealthy system is

---

Box 6.6 **Simple examples of distraction or skewing of attention.**

1 A nurse, carefully calming a distressed patient while adjusting a drip, finds herself called away to the door. There, she is asked to fill in a 'compassion' evaluation questionnaire.
2 'As a GP, I used to see myself as patient-centred. Nowadays, I find myself preoccupied with questions and interventions incentivised by the payment scheme'.
3 'I know that, at the end of my shift, there is always at least an hour's paperwork to process. This makes me rush some of the sensitive, intimate work with patients. I am left feeling that I have been uncaring'.

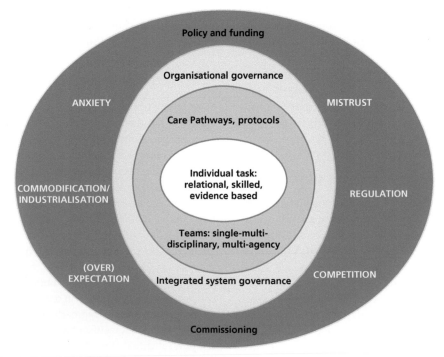

Figure 6.2 The task and role system. Source: Ballatt *et al.* (2020). © 2020, Cambridge University Press.

created. This is more likely to happen if mistrust or fear of blame or sanction is allowed to permeate the system, with everybody 'looking over their shoulders' to fend off danger to their reputation or even jobs (see Box 6.7).

A healthy 'relational' system

Of course, no system is perfect. However carefully leaders try to design and lead an organisation to enable synergy, collaboration and focus on care, there will be mismatches, fault lines and inadequacies. The work will always be costly to practitioners, and there will always be anxiety, about task, and the adequacy of a service. The key is to cultivate a *relational system* within which these realities can be managed constructively and healthily to support humane, collaborative and effective work. Attention must be given to the *psychosocial dynamics* – in the individual's engagement with patients, in the teams in which they work, in the relationships between teams and services and in inter-organisational relationships. It is important that staff be encouraged to value and attend to these matters, and also be given the time and space to address them. The various levels

of attention required are illustrated in Figure 6.3 – again, the task is to address each level individually and all as a whole system.

This system of relationships is, like the task and role system, always vulnerable. Unhealthy dynamics, serious 'malfunctions', can emerge in the face of anxiety, stress, poorly managed inter-professional relationships, competing priorities and uncertainty. The same 'environmental' factors that can lead to a poorly functioning task and role system can harm the relational system, and are, again, indicated in the outer circle. The figure shows both the relationships that are involved for individuals (above the horizontal line) and the team and wider system relationships that require attention (below the line). All aspects of this picture are important to staff well-being, but how staff experience the teams in which they work is especially vital to their well-being and resilience (see Box 6.8).

Conclusion

If staff experience a sense of safety and containment, acknowledgement of their experience and perspectives, and support and encouragement, their well-being will be promoted and sustained. Cultivating a system that generates such felt experience requires attending to potentially destructive, even toxic, dynamics. Leaders, at all levels, but especially at the frontline, need an understanding of these matters, and the skills to address them. This should be seen as a 'duty of care'. They need to develop a 'bifocal view' that bears both the task and role and the relational system in mind. They need skills in building and sustaining healthy teamwork. Space for team, and inter-team, dialogue and reflective practice must be seen and validated as vital aspects of the work. There is a rich tradition of thinking about the characteristics of, and the factors that promote or hinder, healthy teams and systems, including the work of Haigh (2004); West (2017); and Roberts and Obholzer (1994). References

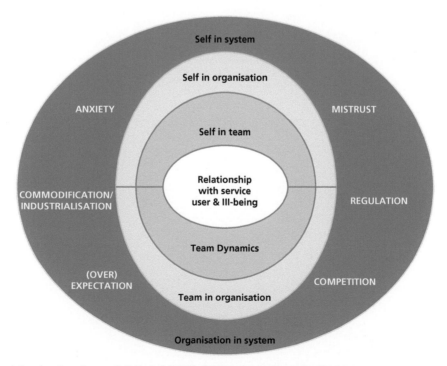

Figure 6.3 The 'kinship' or relational system. Source: Ballatt *et al.* (2020). © 2020, Cambridge University Press.

Box 6.8 **Five qualities of a therapeutic environment, presented as a developmental sequence.**

Quality	Expression in a therapeutic environment
Attachment	A culture of belonging, in which attention is given to joining and leaving, and staff are encouraged to feel as part of a team
Containment	A culture of safety, in which there is a secure organisational structure, and staff feel supported, looked after and cared about within the team
Communication	A culture of openness, in which difficulties and conflict can be voiced, and staff have a reflective, questioning attitude to the work
Involvement	A 'living–learning' culture, in which team members appreciate each other's contributions and have a sense that their work and perspective are valued
Agency	A culture of empowerment, in which all members of the team have a say in the running of the place and play a part in decision-making

Source: Haigh (2004). © 2004, Royal College of Psychiatrists.

to some of these resources are included in the 'Further reading/ resources' section. 'Intelligent kindness' offers an exploration of many of them.

Critical to the challenge is leaders' ability to manage their own anxiety, to remain open to the experience of staff and to work intelligently to manage the potentially damaging effects of unmanaged anxiety in the system. If this work is undertaken well, everybody's well-being and resilience will improve. Rather importantly, the working environment will be one that people will want to come to work in, with consequent improvements in recruitment and retention.

Further reading/resources

Ballatt, J., Campling, P. and Maloney, C. (2020) *Intelligent Kindness: Rehabilitating the Welfare State*. Cambridge University Press, Cambridge, UK.

Bohart, A.C. and Tallman, K. (1999) *How Clients Make Therapy Work: The Process of Active Self-Healing*. American Psychological Association, Washington DC.

Bowlby, J. (1969) *Attachment*. Penguin, London, England.

Haigh, R. (2004) The quintessence of an effective team: some developmental dynamics for staff groups, in *From Toxic Institutions to Therapeutic Environments* (eds P. Campling and R. Haigh, pp. 119–130). Royal College of Psychiatrists, London, UK.

Obholzer, A. and Roberts, V. (1994) *The Unconscious at Work*. Brunner-Routledge, London, UK.

Rendelmeir, D.A., Molin, J. and Tibshirani, R.J. (1995) A randomised trial of compassionate care for the homeless in an emergency department. *Lancet*, **345**, 1131–1134.

Schön, D.A. (1983) *The Reflective Practitioner: How Professionals Think in Action*. Basic Books, London, UK.

Sinclair, S. (1997) *Making Doctors*. Berg Publishers, London, UK.

Weinman, J., Ebrecht, M., Scott, S., *et al.* (2008) Enhanced wound healing after emotional disclosure intervention. *British Journal of Health Psychology*, **13**, 95–102.

West, M. (2017) Collaborative and Compassionate Leadership. Available at: https://www.kingsfund.org.uk/audio-video/michael-west-collaborative-compassionate-leadership (accessed 12.08.2020).

CHAPTER 7

Kindness in Healthcare Teams

Anna Frain

University of Nottingham, Graduate Entry Medical School, Derby Speciality Training Programme for General Practice, UK

Overview

- Kindness in the workplace increases longevity, and improves performance, empathy and creativity.
- Treating colleagues with civility saves patient lives.
- Even small amounts of rudeness in teams adversely affects clinical performance and patient care.
- Schwartz Rounds help build teamwork.
- Managing toxic emotions in the workplace is an essential requirement for building resilient individuals and teams.
- Effective leadership in teams involves intelligent kindness.

'I've learned that people will forget what you said, forget what you did, but people will never forget how you made them feel'.

– Maya Angelou

Introduction

Evidence suggests that team-based working improves efficiency and innovation in patient care; increases staff mental well-being; reduces hospitalisation, clinical errors, violence and aggression towards staff; and lowers patient mortality (Markiewicz *et al.*, 2017).

Kindness is defined as the 'quality of being friendly, generous and considerate'. A kind, resilient, well-functioning healthcare team provides optimal patient care, resulting in improved clinical outcomes. The term 'caring profession' is used to describe those working in all aspects of healthcare. The care at the centre of our teams should extend to each other and ourselves, as well as to our patients.

Understanding and communication between professionals is a key part of teamwork. As professionals in modern healthcare, we cannot care for our patients alone. We depend on each other as members of the healthcare team.

In this chapter, we address ways in which teams can flourish and succeed with kindness at their core. We also see that dysfunctional teams, where care is disrupted by individuals or poor leadership, results in negative outcomes for patients. We will also consider how this toxicity in the clinical environment can be identified, addressed and reversed.

Kindness in teams

'Cure sometimes, treat often and comfort always'.

– Hippocrates.

Kindness is essential in healthcare. There is clear evidence that patient safety depends on kindness. What happened in the Mid Staffordshire Trust in the UK (see Chapter 8) was described as 'a chilling indictment of what happens when we lose sight of the importance of kindness when caring for our patients' (Mathers, 2016). Mathers goes on to say: 'it is kindness which makes us human, builds resilience, and makes us better doctors and better people'. Treating colleagues with respect and appreciation makes them twice as likely to act in the same way towards someone else (www.civilitysaveslives.com).

Our professionalism requires us to treat those in our care with respect. This needs to be extended to our colleagues. Some of the benefits of kindness in the workplace are outlined by Chancellor *et al.* (2017). They discuss the impact of pro-social behaviour (doing kind acts for others) and its implications for the workplace (see Box 7.1). There is evidence that staff well-being predicts outcomes that include better performance, reliable work, persistence and better feedback. Pro-social behaviour buffers staff against burnout and emotional exhaustion, and promotes perspective,

---

Box 7.1 **Georgia's jar of coffee.**

Georgia, a receptionist, sent an instant message offering Anna, a GP, a cup of coffee. However, she then realised there was no decaffeinated coffee (which Anna always drank), and sent a message of apology.

The following day, Anna was surprised to have a cup of decaffeinated coffee on her desk. She discovered that Georgia had been shopping with her Mum the night before, bought a jar of decaffeinated coffee and dropped it in to the practice on her day off.

Anna felt touched by Georgia's kindness and thoughtfulness. This meant far more to her than a jar of coffee.

---

empathy and creativity. A study by Shirom *et al.* (2011) showed that the positive support of co-workers increased longevity.

Clare Gerada, a UK GP working with struggling professionals, promotes teamwork as part of the way we guard ourselves against burnout. Her 'B.U.R.N.O.U.T.' acronym can be seen in Box 7.2.

Schwartz Rounds (see the following text) may help us to understand each other and our roles, and thereby appreciate the stress we feel and help us understand what might help us improve our work.

Guidelines on how to communicate clearly include effective ways to disseminate important clinical advice and guidelines within a team, ensuring everyone receives the information they need.

The simple but effective concept of 'most respectful interpretation' is explored in Chapter 9, which, when used in teams, can help reduce misunderstanding and miscommunication.

Civility

The campaign civilitysaveslives.com in the UK states:

> '*A medical environment where staff are good to each other is a safer one. And there is research to back it up*'.

Chris Turner, the consultant in emergency medicine who started the campaign in 2018, points out that kindness is a virtue, but civility, which comes up repeatedly in research, is central to professionalism and is a behaviour. We can consciously change how we behave, and his campaign gives a clear positive message. He came to the realisation that, although process is necessary, people were the most important part of a team. Box 7.3 shows some reflections on civility in teams.

Kelli Harding, in her book *The Rabbit Effect* (2019), explores the effect of kindness on health. She describes how relationships, especially those at work, particularly considering the significant amount of time we spend there, impact our health. In the 'rabbit studies', kindness changed the outcome in a way not previously envisaged. Her experience in medicine confirmed that relationships with colleagues and the feeling that you are supported as a person had a beneficial effect on performance and well-being. Simple things – such as asking a colleague how their weekend was, checking that they are OK or taking a short break with a colleague – have been found to boost a community at work.

Effects of rudeness and incivility

Small amounts of rudeness cause significant effects on cognitive performance (Porath and Erez, 2011). This includes creative tasks and helpfulness, affecting the recipient as well as witnesses. Just being around an uncivil environment has a negative effect on people (see Box 7.4).

In a healthcare team, both staff and patients are affected by incivility. They may be unable to ask for help or feel anxious. Staff may not realise that they and/or the team are underperforming nor recognise the gravity of the situation.

Chris Turner (www.civilitysaveslives) suggests that we should both call out incivility when we witness it and become more self-aware of when we instigate it ourselves (see Figure 7.1). We should develop and promote an alternative culture of active kindness.

Riskin *et al.* (2015) found that even small amounts of perceived rudeness affects the recipient, the bystanders and patient outcomes. Their trial in a simulated paediatric environment demonstrated shocking detrimental effects on whole teams. In 2019, Katz *et al.* showed that incivility had negative impacts on staff vigilance, diagnosis, communication and patient management.

Kindness in leadership

> '*I suppose leadership at one time meant muscles, but today it means getting along with people*'.
> – Mahatma Gandhi

Box 7.2 B.U.R.N.O.U.T. – An acronym to prevent burnout.

- **B**alance work and play – between the machinery of caring and actual caring, declutter the space in the consulting room between us and our patients.
- **U**nderstand our limitations – we are not superheroes.
- **R**ecognise – prevent and treat burnout in ourselves and our teams.
- **N**urture the next generation.
- **T**eamwork – working in groups, restore the times and spaces to work, rest, play and reflect together.

Source: Gerada (2017). © 2017, Clare Gerada.

Box 7.3 Civility in teams.

Almost all excellence in healthcare is dependent on teams, and teams work best when all members feel safe and have a voice.

Civility between team members creates that sense of safety and is a key ingredient of great teams.

Incivility robs teams of their potential.

Source: Civility Saves Lives. © 2020, www.civilitysaveslives.com.

Box 7.4 Effects of incivility on workers.

Workers on the receiving end of incivility:
- 48% intentionally decreased their work effort
- 47% intentionally decreased the time spent at work
- 38% intentionally decreased the quality of their work
- 80% lost work time worrying about the incident
- 63% lost work time avoiding the offender
- 66% said their performance declined
- 78% said their commitment to the organisation declined
- 12% said they had left their job because of the uncivil treatment
- 25% admitted to taking out their frustration on customers.

Source: Porath and Pearson (2013). © 2013, Harvard Business School Publishing.

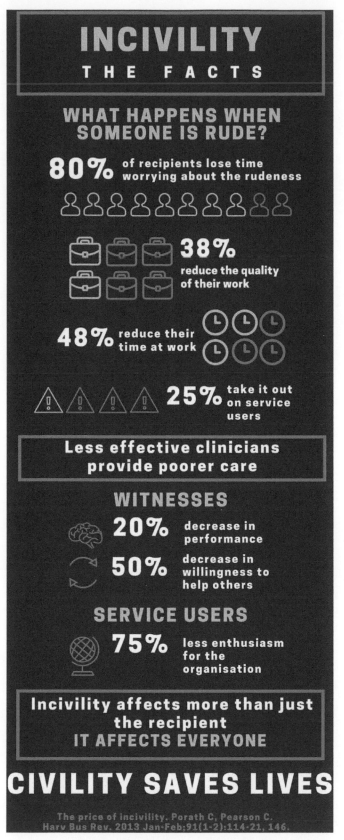

Figure 7.1 Incivility the facts poster. Source: Chris Turner / Civility Saves Lives.

Clinical leadership refers to the concept of healthcare professionals undertaking leadership tasks such as setting goals and promoting values for their team. Their clinical background helps to ground everything with the patient at the centre.

The NHS Leadership Academy outlines how we can lead teams in providing care. This includes providing a caring safe environment to enable everyone to do their job properly. Leaders should essentially be:

- *caring* for the team
- *proficient* in recognising underlying reasons for behaviour
- *strong* in providing opportunities for mutual support
- *exemplary* in spreading a caring environment.

In 2018, Smith *et al.* (2018) concluded that supportive nurse managers reduce co-worker incivility. Christine Porath showed that what people wanted mostly was to be treated with respect by their leaders. Thanking people, sharing credit, listening attentively, humbly asking questions and smiling helped to achieve this (see Box 7.5).

Communication in teams

Communication between ourselves in front of patients influences the care we provide to them. Treating each other, as well as those for whom we care, with respect improves clinical outcomes. Communication between team members away from patients is also important.

Clinicians themselves describe being affected by sub-optimal communication and a lack of kindness. Their stories indicate ways we can, as healthcare teams, improve outcomes for our patients.

Kieran Sweeny, a GP, was diagnosed with mesothelioma. His experiences explain the effects on the patient of thoughtless communication and the inability of a team to speak honestly with the patient. It reminds us how vital honest, clear, compassionate care is to patients' progress (see Box 7.6).

Kate Granger also experienced life as a patient and promoted compassionate care. Simple issues – for example, not even introducing ourselves, led her to comment:

> 'We run wards for the convenience of our staff, not for the benefit of our patients'.
>
> – Dr Kate Granger, 'Hello my name is. . .'

Box 7.5 **Compassionate governance.**

Respect the team. Civility saves lives.
Respect complexity. No instant conclusions.
Look at all outcomes. Especially the great.
Accept errors are inevitable. Learn from them.
Facilitate people changing themselves.

Source: Based on Civility Saves Lives. www.civilitysaveslives.com.

Box 7.6 **Effects of poor communication – lack of kindness – on patients.**

Medicine is about understanding and being with people at the edge of the human predicament'.
  'Clinicians inadvertently heap small humiliations on patients'.
  'I felt humiliated. I felt utterly degraded'.
  'Rediscovering the humanity in a patient. . . That is why I came into medicine'.
  Only serious people can be healthcare professionals as it is a deadly serious profession'.

Source: Dr Kieran Sweeney (YouTube, 2012)

Kate started the campaign 'Hello my name is. . .', which showed that kindness could start with something as simple as ensuring the patient knows who we are and our roles. During a difficult hospital admission she had, Kate describes the porter as being the only person who asked her how she was feeling and listened to her. Her husband Chris said:

> *She said you should always see the patient as though he or she were one of your relatives, because then you would take extra care with them and go above and beyond what a person would expect'.*

A healthcare team aware of the problems encountered by Dr Sweeney and Dr Grainger can transform the experience of patients. An inclusive team, recognising every member from the porter to the physiotherapist, consultant, nurse and receptionist, can provide better treatment for their patients (see Box 7.7).

Schwartz Rounds

In 1994, Ken Schwartz was diagnosed with terminal lung cancer. He found that simple acts of kindness from his caregivers 'made the unbearable bearable'. He left a legacy for the establishment of the Schwartz Centre in Boston to help foster compassion in healthcare.

Box 7.7 **Training in a team.**

During the annual safeguarding training in a general practice, non-clinical and clinical team members work in inter-professional teams. They discuss cases and learn from each other. They understand that the receptionist can recognise a red flag, such as the behaviour of a parent to a child in the waiting room, or the fact a father rings to ask for an appointment for a teenager with vaginal discharge. This concern or red flag is passed on to the clinician, especially the safeguarding lead, and this highlights the need for extra care to be taken.
  Children will be safer in a practice where everyone works together, appreciating each other's perspective and where the culture is to listen to each other and be approachable.

> *'I have learned that medicine is not merely about performing tests or surgeries, or administering drugs. . . For as skilled and knowledgeable as my caregivers are, what matters most is that they have empathised with me in a way that gives me hope and makes me feel like a human being and not just an illness'.*

Schwartz Rounds developed in the USA in the late 1990s and were first introduced in the UK in 2011. They aim to provide a forum for healthcare professionals to explore some of the challenging emotional and psychosocial issues resulting from patient care. Regular monthly or fortnightly rounds enable different professionals to share their experiences in a safe, confidential environment. Concentrating on the emotional impact rather than clinical decisions and outcomes encourages reflection rather than problem-solving.

The rounds include clinical and non-clinical staff and focus on understanding experience from a social and emotional point of view. They are not a form of clinical supervision or debriefing. The round lasts an hour, and starts with three staff sharing their experience for 15 minutes and then a facilitator leading an open discussion. In the UK, the pilot rounds varied from an average of 30–95 participants. You can see one in action (see the 'Further reading/resources' section).

The Kings Fund (Goodrich, 2011) reports that Schwartz Rounds have demonstrated a need and are greatly valued by staff who participate (70% rating of excellence). Participants felt that teamwork was strengthened by encouraging networking, improving multidisciplinary working and fostering better understanding and co-operation.

> *'Anecdotally, nursing staff, physios, all staff, really, say they have a greater sympathy for doctors who seem less cold and hard. And doctors have greater respect for the rest of the team as you appreciate what they do and what they are having to take home with them'.*

Smith *et al.* (2020) showed that second-year medical students who engaged fully and understood the process of Schwartz Rounds through facilitation could improve empathy and understanding towards patients and colleagues.

Bullying in the workplace and the toxic individual

Bullying is common. Up to 50% of nurses might experience or witness bullying (Logan and Malone, 2018). Workplace bullying is strongly associated with negative nursing outcomes, including intent to leave, work dissatisfaction and turnover. Bullying is associated with an increase in adverse events for patients, including infections and falls. A Norwegian study of nurses (Olsen *et al.*, 2017) showed that bullying negatively influences job satisfaction and work performance. The UK General Medical Council states that doctors should not bully colleagues but should treat them with respect.

In confronting bullying, the available resources outlined by the Royal College of Emergency Medicine Wellness Compendium (Hewitt and Kennedy, 2020) include the Australasian College of

Emergency Medicine's action plan to investigate allegations of bullying. The blog titled 'Bully for you' suggests that we all participate in bullying at some time. The Royal College of Surgeons' anti-bullying and undermining campaign titled 'Let's remove it' provides evidence of the impact that bullying has on patient safety and the clinical team – for example, healthcare professionals attribute disruptive behaviour in the perioperative area alone to 67% of adverse events, 71% of medical errors and 27% of perioperative deaths (Royal College of Surgeons Edinburgh, 'Let's remove it').

The CanMEDS Physician Health Guide (see the 'Further reading/resources' section) (Puddester *et al.*, 2019) explores, through case histories and resolutions, how and why issues such as intimidation and harassment in training and disruptive professional behaviours might arise. It may be difficult to recognise a toxic individual (see Box 7.8). Action must be taken to mitigate the negative effects of a toxic individual's behaviour; it may, at times, result in the removal of the individual from the team.

Avoiding Toxic workplaces

Establishing a mutually respectful workplace has been explored in a clinical oncology setting by Duma *et al.* (2019), where factors such as harassment, discrimination, unconscious bias, incivility and micro-aggressions are counterbalanced by micro-affirmations, inclusivity, psychological safety, gender equality and legal protection. Building bridges and not barriers between generations, cultures and genders is positive action. Education enables the recognition of microaggression and ensures sustainable, good working relationships. They recommend a shared vision, being prepared to start from scratch, praising individuality, leading by example, creating policies together with all team members and ensuring the well-being and professionalism of all team members. It is challenging to resolve issues in a toxic or exclusive environment and resolution requires organisational as well as team commitment.

Positive factors of jobs (job resources) such as career opportunities, co-worker support, role clarity, participation in decision-making and skill variety can mitigate against job demands such as high work pressure, an unfavourable work environment and emotionally demanding interactions with work colleagues.

Conclusion

Kindness and civility are fundamental to maximising the effectiveness of healthcare teams. Kindness and civility save lives. There is an increasing amount of evidence related to the role of kindness and civility in the provision of safe healthcare. Rudeness and incivility affect not only the victim but other team members, patients and onlookers. In this chapter, we have discussed the effects of rudeness and incivility on patients, which include their feelings of humiliation. Schwartz Rounds were developed following Ken Schwartz' describing kindness as making 'the unbearable bearable'. Bullying and toxic individuals damage teamwork; their behaviour needs recognition and action. Those in leadership positions must recognise negative factors affecting the team as well as acts of kindness. It is reassuring to see evidence increasingly confirming our instinctive feeling that even small acts of kindness and pro-social behaviour can have large positive effects on teams.

'Each time a man stands up for an ideal, or acts to improve the lot of others, or strikes out against injustice, he sends forth a tiny ripple of hope, and crossing each other from a million different centres of energy and daring, those ripples build a current which can sweep down the mightiest walls of oppression and resistance'.

– Robert F. Kennedy

Box 7.8 **Recognising a toxic individual.**

During a tutorial, Saima heard about an incident where the clinical supervisor (CS) became extremely angry with a trainee during a debrief in front of a medical student. The student had already told Saima that this had happened and had been quite upset.

Saima recalled a situation several months earlier when the same CS had become angry with Saima, threatened to refer her to the professional governing body and told her that she was mentally unstable and should resign.

Saima was significantly senior to the CS but felt she could not act due to the threats. It was only when she heard the trainee's experience that she knew she must and immediately did act to protect them.

The whole team, aware of the original incident, then realised that the CS was repeatedly acting as a bully. There were many other issues which should have been recognised, but everyone had failed to act.

They sought advice and took the action required. The CS soon left the organisation.

References

Chancellor, J., Margolis, S., Bao, K.J. and Lyubomirsky, S. (2017) Everyday Prosociality in the workplace. The reinforcing benefits of giving, getting and glimpsing. *Emotion*, **18** (4). DOI: 10.1037/emo0000321.

Duma, N., Maingi, S., Tap, W. *et al.* (2019) Establishing a mutually respectful environment in the workplace: a toolbox for performance excellence. *American Society of Clinical Oncology Educational Book*, **39**, e219–226.

Gerada, C. (2017) *ABC of Clinical Professionalism*. Wiley, London.

Goodrich, J. (2011) *Schwartz Rounds – Evaluation of the UK Pilots*. The Kings Fund. London, UK

Harding, K. (2019) *The Rabbit Effect*. Atria Books, New York, NY.

Hewitt, S. and Kennedy, U. (2020) *The Wellness Compendium*. Royal College of Emergency Medicine, London, UK.

Katz, D., Blasius, K., Isaak, R. *et al.* (2019) Exposure to incivility hinders performance in a simulated operative crisis. *BMJ Quality and Safety*, **28**, 750–757.

Logan, T. and Malone, D.M. (2018) Nurses' perceptions of teamwork and workplace bullying. *Journal of Nurse Management*, **26** (4), 411–419.

Markiewicz, L., West, M. and McKimm, J. (2017) Leading groups and teams (Chapter 5). ABC of Clinical Leadership. BMJ Books, London, UK.

Mathers, N. (2016) Compassion and the science of kindness: Harvard Davis Lecture 2015. *British Journal of General Practice*, **66** (648), e525–e527.

Olsen, E., Bjaalid, G. and Mikkelsen, A. (2017) Work climate and the mediating role of workplace bullying related to job performance, job satisfaction, and work ability: A study among hospital nurses. *Journal Advances Nursing*, **73** (11), 2709–2719.

Porath, C. and Erez, A. (2011) How rudeness takes its toll. *British Psychological Society*, **24**, 508–511.

Porath, C. and Pearson, C. (2013) The price of incivility. *Harvard Business Review*, **91** (1–2), 114–121, 146.

Puddester, D., Flynn, L. and Cohen, J. (2019) *CanMEDS Physician Health Guide: A Practical Handbook for Physician Health and Well-being.* The Royal College of Physicians and Surgeons of Canada, Ottawa.

Riskin, A., Erez, A. and Foulk, T.A. (2015). The impact of rudeness on medical team performance: a randomised trial. *Paediatrics*, **136** (3), 487–495.

Shirom, A., Toker, S., Alaky, Y. *et al.* (2011) Work-based predictions of mortality: a 20 year follow up of healthy employees. *Health Psychology*, **30** (3), 268–275.

Smith, J., Stewart, M., Foggin, S. *et al.* (2020) Schwartz Centre Rounds in second-year medical students using clinical educator-facilitator group work session: not just 'a facilitated moan"! *BMC Medical Education*, **20**, 271.

Smith, J.G., Morin, K.H. and Lake, E.T. (2018) Association of the nurse work environment with nurse incivility in hospitals. *Journal of Nurse Management*, **26** (2), 219–226.

Further reading/resources

Arnetz, J., Fitzpatrick, L., Cotton, S. *et al.* (2019) Workplace bullying among nurses: developing a model for intervention. *Violence and Victims*, **34** (2).

Cracknell, A. and Cooper, N. (2017) Communication in teams (Chapter 5). *ABC of Clinical Communication.* BMJ Books.

Peachy, R. (2020) Tackling toxic tribalism in the health care service. *National Health Executive.*

Porath, C. (2016) *Mastering Civility. A Manifesto for the Workplace.* New York.

Porath, C. (2018) *Why Being Respectful to Your Co-workers is Good for Business.* TED talks, University of Nevada.

Swanwick, T. and McKimm, J. (2017) *ABC of Clinical Leadership.* BMJ Books, Wiley, London, UK.

Turner, C. (2019) *When Rudeness in Teams Turns Deadly.* TED Talks. TEDx Exeter.

Wald, H.S. (2020) Optimizing resilience and well-being for healthcare professions trainees and healthcare professionals during public health crises – Practical tips for an 'integrative resilience' approach, *Medical Teacher*, **42** (7), 744–755.

Websites

Civility Saves Lives. Available at: civilitysaveslives.com.

hellomynameis. Available at: https://www.hellomynameis.org.uk The Point of Foundation Care. Available at: www.pointofcarefoundation.org.uk/resource/dr-kieran-sweeney-talks-experiences-cancer-patient/ (accessed 11.01.2021).

Regarding Schwartz Rounds. Available at: www.thepointofcarefoundation.org.uk (accessed 11/1/2021).

The Nine Leadership Dimensions. Available at: https://www.leadershipacademy.nhs.uk/resources/healthcare-leadership-model/nine-leadership-dimensions/ (accessed 11/1/2021).

Watch a Schwartz Round. Available at: www.pointofcarefoundation.org.uk/resource/watch-a-schwartz-round/ (last accessed 11/10/2020).

Wellness Compendium. Available at: https://www.rcem.ac.uk/docs/SustainableWorking

CHAPTER 8

Organisational Kindness

Nicola Cooper[1,2] and Barry Evans[2]

[1] Medical Education Centre, University of Nottingham, UK
[2] University Hospitals of Derby & Burton NHS Foundation Trust, UK

OVERVIEW

- 'Moral injury' is a term which acknowledges the fact that resilience and burnout are always contextual.

- Organisational kindness exists at four levels: the individual; groups and teams; healthcare organisations; and the wider system.

- A kind healthcare organisation has three main roles in relation to its staff: that of an interface with the wider healthcare system; of optimising its resources; and of maintaining the organisation's reputation and values.

- For patient safety to be maintained, staff must have the confidence that their organisation will respond to their concerns.

- Employee motivation is determined by 'hygiene factors' and 'motivators', which in turn influence productivity and performance.

Introduction

Resilience is the capacity to recover quickly from difficulties; it protects us from burnout. While we all know what the term 'burnout' conveys, it has, in fact, no standard definition. The term was coined in the 1970s by Freudenberger to describe a constellation of symptoms – malaise, fatigue, frustration, cynicism, and inefficacy – that arise from making excessive demands on energy, strength or resources in the workplace. Rather than a single disorder, burnout is really a spectrum of symptoms, affecting up to 40% of UK doctors and nurses. The Maslach Burnout Inventory has been used for the past few decades to quantify burnout (see Figure 8.1). The Word Health Organization International Classification of Diseases defines burnout as 'a state of vital exhaustion'.

For more than a decade, the term *burnout* has been used to describe clinician distress. This had its problems: it implied perhaps that something was wrong with clinicians who suffered from burnout, that they were somehow deficient compared with their (possibly) more resilient colleagues. Resilience training was introduced by healthcare organisations. However, resilience and burnout are always contextual. In 2018, the conversation about clinician distress shifted to the concept of 'moral injury'. Moral injury was first described in Vietnam War veterans who had symptoms similar to that of post-traumatic stress disorder – only, instead of experiencing imminent threats to their personal safety, they had experienced repeated insults to their personal morality. They had been forced, in some way, to act contrary to what their beliefs held to be right (see Figure 8.2).

As clinicians, we take seriously our duty to put patients first. A career in healthcare is often seen as a calling rather than a job, involving a degree of devotion, sacrifice and long hours. The first duty of a doctor, according to the UK's General Medical Council, is: 'Make the care of your patient your first concern' (see Figure 8.3). Every time we are forced to make a decision that seems to contravene our patients' best interests, we feel a sense of moral injustice. Over time, these repetitive insults amount to moral injury. Moral injury describes the challenge of simultaneously knowing what patients need but being unable to provide it due to constraints that are seemingly beyond our control.

Talbot and Dean (2019; see the 'Further reading/resources' section) state: 'We have come to believe that burnout is the end stage of moral injury, when clinicians are physically and emotionally exhausted with battling a broken system in their efforts to provide good care; when they feel ineffective because too often they have met with immovable barriers to good care; and when they depersonalise patients because emotional investment is intolerable when patient suffering is inevitable as a result of system dysfunction'. Talking about moral injury, as opposed to burnout, shifts attention to the broken system.

The effects of moral injury

When clinicians are *exhausted* with battling a broken system, they give up as a means of self-preservation. The clinician's voice – canaries in the coalmine of healthcare – is lost. This eventually results in the opposite of quality: unsafe, inefficient and ineffective healthcare.

When clinicians *feel ineffective* because they are usually met with immovable barriers to good care, the result is a sense of betrayal and mistrust. The breach of a person's ethical code at the heart of moral injury can inflict lasting behavioural, emotional and psychological damage, distorting a person's self-identity and provoking a reflexive distrust of others. This eventually results in a lack of clinical leadership, which in turn has a negative impact on patient outcomes (see the case history in Box 8.1).

ABC of Clinical Resilience, First Edition. Edited by Anna Frain, Sue Murphy, and John Frain.
© 2021 John Wiley & Sons Ltd. Published 2021 by John Wiley & Sons Ltd.

The MBI is a validated psychological inventory consisting of 22 items relating to occupational burnout. It measures three dimensions: emotional exhaustion, depersonalisation and personal accomplishment. The MBI takes 10–15 minutes to complete and can be administered to individuals or groups.

Emotional Exhaustion

The nine-item emotional exhaustion scale measures feelings of being emotionally overextended and exhausted at one's work. Higher scores correspond to greater experienced burnout.

Depersonalisation

The five-item depersonalisation scale measures an unfeeling and impersonal response toward recipients of one's service, care, treatment or instruction. Higher scores correspond to greater degrees of experienced burnout.

Personal accomplishment

The eight-item personal accomplishment scale measures feelings of competence and successful achievement in one's work with people. Lower scores correspond to greater experienced burnout.

Figure 8.1 Maslach Burnout Inventory (MBI). Source: Adapted from Maslach *et al.* (1996–2016).

Military example	Healthcare example
Military personnel are highly trained professionals prepared to enter conflict zones and face violence, injury and even death. The 'military covenant' is an unwritten promise by a nation to ensure that those who serve, and their families, will be treated fairly.	Healthcare personnel are highly trained professionals prepared to work in challenging environments that may, at times, put their own safety at risk. The NHS Constitution for England sets out the principles and values of the NHS, including the NHS' pledges to its staff..
The Iraq War in 2003, in which a US-led coalition overthrew the government of Saddam Hussain, was based on the alleged presence of weapons of mass destruction in the country, which were never found. Many NATO countries opposed the war, and the secretary general of the United Nations declared the war illegal. UK troops, hailed as heroes, suffered from a lack of protective equipment, and many died. More than 1000 cases of alleged war crimes were filed against British military personnel by one UK solicitor, who was subsequently struck off. All but one of the charges were dropped several years later.	The COVID-19 pandemic first peaked in the UK in May 2020. The UK government had failed to act on recommendations from a pandemic preparation exercise, code-named 'Operation Cygnus', in 2016, during a period of economic austerity. UK healthcare workers, hailed as heroes, suffered from a lack of protective equipment at the start of the pandemic. All 'routine' care was postponed to free up capacity, including urgent cancer investigations and treatments. Hospital and care home visits were banned, meaning that patients died of COVID-19 without their loved ones being able to visit.
Following these events, there was a debate about the military covenant in the UK, covering issues as diverse as protective equipment, housing, pay, protection from malicious prosecution and access to healthcare for veterans, including mental healthcare.	During this period, much was unknown about this new disease, its clinical presentations and transmission. Public health messaging appeared confusing. There was a debate about the value that society places on key workers such as nurses, covering issues as diverse as protective equipment, pay and being charged to park at their place of work.

Figure 8.2 Moral injury: the challenge of simultaneously knowing what is right and what is needed, but being unable to provide it due to constraints seemingly beyond our control. Source: Based on Armed Forces Covenant, proudly supporting those who serve. https://www.armedforcescovenant.gov.uk/.

When clinicians *depersonalise patients* because emotional investment is intolerable as a result of system dysfunction, the result is a lack of person-centred care and maybe a lack of care for others in the team. This eventually results in a cycle of dissatisfaction and poor care.

It is not enough to look at individuals, and other resources need to be explored which can act as levers through which organisational kindness can simultaneously reduce the impact of moral injury and burnout and improve outcomes for patients.

Levels of organisational kindness

Strategies that focus on individuals alone to improve quality are seldom effective. Healthcare is delivered by individuals who work in groups and teams within healthcare organisations, which in turn are part of a wider system. The greatest impact can be achieved by considering all four levels simultaneously (see Figure 8.4).

The interface with the wider healthcare system

Healthcare organisations exist as the interface between groups and teams of people and the wider healthcare system. Core to organisational kindness is organisational leadership and organisational culture. *Organisational culture* has been defined as 'A set of basic tacit assumptions about how the world is and ought to be that is shared by a set of people and determines their perceptions, thoughts and feelings, and ... behaviour' (Schein, 1985; see the 'Further reading/resources' section). These values, beliefs and behaviours are reflected in 'how we do things around here'.

Patients must be able to trust doctors with their lives and health. To justify that trust, you must show respect for human life and make sure your practice meets the standards expected of you in four domains.

Knowledge, skills and performance

- Make the care of your patient your first concern
- Provide a good standard of practice and care
  - Keep your professional knowledge and skills up to date
  - Recognise and work within the limits of your competence

Safety and quality

- Take prompt action if you think that patient safety, dignity or comfort is being compromised
- Protect and promote the health of patients and the public

Communication, partnership and teamwork

- Treat patients as individuals, and respect their dignity
  - Treat patients politely and considerately
  - Respect patients' right to confidentiality
- Work in partnership with patients
  - Listen to, and respond to, their concerns and preferences
  - Give patients the information they want or need in a way that they can understand
  - Respect patients' right to reach decisions with you about their treatment and care
  - Support patients in caring for themselves to improve and maintain their health
- Work with colleagues in ways that best serve patients' interests
- Maintain trust
- Be honest and open, and act with integrity
- Never discriminate unfairly against patients or colleagues
- Never abuse your patients' trust in you or the public's trust in the profession

You are personally accountable for your professional practice and must always be prepared to justify your decisions and actions.

Figure 8.3 General Medical Council Duties of a Doctor. Source: General Medical Council (2019). © 2020, GMC.

Box 8.1 **Development of moral injury in a clinician.**

In 2011, before the Francis Inquiry report* was published, Dr X was the clinical lead of a modern, newly configured department of medicine in a large hospital. In response to pressure from the Department of Health over the 4-hour emergency standard (waiting times in the emergency department), the chief executive decided that patients waiting for a bed would wait in holding areas owned by the receiving department. Although this proposal was meant to be temporary and drive improvements in patient flow downstream, the result was long lines of patients on the admission unit corridor and no additional staff to care for them. Patients frequently deteriorated and even died on the corridor. Ward rounds were conducted on the corridor or in offices where patients occasionally slept on camp beds. Patients even contacted the local newspaper from time to time to come and take photographs of the corridor. Despite all Dr X's suggestions to improve patient flow, incident reports and warnings about safety at every level, the response of senior managers was to do nothing. In fact, there was a joke that they knew things were bad when Dr X started e-mailing photographs of the corridor. Dr X, a hard-working and creative clinical leader, soon began to feel depressed as a result of moral injury. Dr X eventually left, but the sense of betrayal and distrust lingered – and, although she eventually recovered, she never worked in a clinical leadership role again.

*The Francis Inquiry report was published on 6 February 2013 and examined the causes of the gross failings in care at Mid Staffordshire NHS Foundation Trust between 2005 and 2009.

Level	Examples
Individual	Education
	Training
	Data feedback
	Leadership development
Group/team	Task redesign
	Collaboration
	Guidelines, procedures, pathways
	Team development
Organisation	Organisational culture
	Organisational learning
	Organisational development
	Continuous improvement/total quality management
Wider system	Government policies
	Payment systems
	National bodies
	Evidence-based practice knowledge centres

Figure 8.4 Four levels of change. Source: Adapted from Ferlie and Shortell (2001).

The healthcare organisation has an opportunity to shape the culture in which staff work. Examples of how organisations can facilitate a culture of kindness include recent work on incivility in the workplace and its impact on performance in healthcare organisations (see the 'Further reading/resources' section). This has led to the 'Civility Saves Lives' campaign, in which we are exhorted to replace rudeness by a kinder, more effective – and ultimately safer – way of communication (see Figure 8.5).

In its interface role, the organisation must deliver targets set by the wider system, but also respond to the concerns and ideas expressed by groups and individuals, which includes patients and carers as well as staff. When an organisation fails to do this, it can lead to long-term harm – as manifest in a series of widely publicised scandals in the UK such as that which led to the Mid Staffordshire NHS Foundation Trust Public Enquiry in 2012.

The Berwick Report (see the 'Further reading/resources' section) explicitly describes the need for organisations to 'Embrace transparency unequivocally and everywhere in the service of accountability, trust and the growth of knowledge'. However, in order to raise concerns, staff must have the confidence that their organisation will respond in a kind and compassionate manner, free of retribution. The report also describes the need for regulatory bodies to 'Be respectful of the goodwill and sound intention of the vast majority of staff', but include a hierarchy of responses, including recourse to criminal sanctions as a rare deterrent for wilful or reckless neglect or mistreatment.

Compassionate leadership is being championed by NHS Improvement, the organisation that supports the NHS in improving care for patients. While the word 'compassionate' might conjure up ideas of weak leadership, in fact the opposite is true. As Don Berwick, President Emeritus and Senior Fellow of The Institute for Healthcare Improvement, explained:

'Compassionate leadership requires courage. The courage to listen to tough messages from those we lead. The courage to explore their understanding of the challenges they face and to have our own interpretations challenged and rejected. The courage to feel how draining it is to work a 70-hour week, to not have time to go to the toilet on a shift, to have no access to food and drink on a night shift, or to be on the receiving end of violence or abuse from members of the public. And the courage to accept that practicing compassionate leadership will first and foremost address the most apparently intractable workplace challenges such as excessive workload, staff shortages and ever-increasing demand'.

When someone is rude:

- 80% of recipients lose time worrying about the rudeness
- 48% reduce their time at work
- 38% reduce the quality of their work
- 25% take it out on service users

Less effective clinicians provide poorer care: *civility saves lives*.

Figure 8.5 The price of incivility. Source: Adapted from Civility Saves Lives. www.civilitysaveslives.com.

Optimising resources

In addition to serving as an interface, a key responsibility of any healthcare organisation is to use its resources effectively. These resources can be divided into four categories:

- *Finances*: For example, recent funding was made available to enhance staff spaces and rest facilities for junior doctors in the NHS. Providing basic front-line equipment needed for patient care (e.g., desk space, computers, personal protective equipment) through efficient and cost-effective procurement processes is another example of effective resource use that supports staff.
- *Processes* (e.g., embedded practices and technological support): For example, processes that make it easy for staff to 'do the right thing' and provide safe and effective care are important. In many healthcare settings, processes may not be fit for purpose. Involving front-line staff in continuous quality improvement is vital. Likewise, ensuring information technology supports rather than frustrates clinical processes is another example of using resources effectively in a way that supports staff.
- *Places*: Poor working environments can lead to frustration and fatigue. Ensuring a physically and psychologically safe and well-maintained environment, with staff spaces for breaks and education/training, directly contributes to staff well-being.
- *People* (e.g., staff, patients, carers): Investing in resources to support personal and professional development and career progression leads to motivated staff who feel supported in their role and incentivised to 'go the extra mile' when required by their organisation.

Maintaining the organisation's reputation and values

As long ago as the 1960s, psychologist Frederick Herzberg sought to find elements that motivated people at work. His findings have been scrutinised by others – and, with the transition to the knowledge economy, new factors have emerged, but his work is still influential today. Job satisfaction and job dissatisfaction are not opposites. People have two sets of needs – 'hygiene needs', influenced by the physical and physiological conditions at the workplace, and 'motivational needs', tied to the nature of the work itself (see Figure 8.6).

The kind organisation focuses on both sets of needs using its resources effectively to address sources of job dissatisfaction and motivation – which in turn improve productivity and performance.

Hygiene factors (factors for dissatisfaction)	Motivators (factors for satisfaction)
Organisational policies	Achievement
Supervision	Recognition
Relationship with supervisor	The work itself
Work conditions	Responsibility
Status	Advancement
Security	Growth
Pay	

Figure 8.6 Herzberg's hygiene factors and motivators. Source: Adapted from Herzberg (2003).

The effect of kindness on employees can include happiness and motivation, but kindness also impacts on the reputation of an organisation, attracting talent which can in turn create a positive spiral of cultural improvement, derived from relationships formed from an ever-improving people resource.

Unfortunately, even the kindest healthcare organisations cannot mitigate the impact of re-organisations. Frequent re-organisations, as experienced in many healthcare systems despite lack of evidence for their effectiveness in terms of finances or patient care, can harm relationships, create anxiety and lead to 'A loss of momentum, some significant risks of harm to staff and risks of creating cynicism, particularly among clinicians' (Edwards, 2010; see the 'Further reading/resources' section). Due to external forces, even the kindest organisations can inadvertently find themselves returning to conditions that create moral injury among healthcare professionals.

Improving joy at work

The Institute of Healthcare Improvement has gone one step further with the publication of its 2017 white paper 'IHI framework for improving joy at work' (Perlo *et al.*, 2017):

> 'With increasing demands on time, resources, and energy, in addition to poorly designed systems, it's not surprising health care professionals are experiencing burnout at increasingly higher rates, with staff turnover rates also on the rise. Yet, joy in work is more than just the absence of burnout or an issue of individual wellness; it is a system property.
>
> Burnout leads to lower levels of staff engagement, patient experience, and productivity, and an increased risk of workplace accidents. Lower levels of staff engagement are linked with lower-quality patient care, including safety, and burnout limits providers' empathy – a crucial component of effective and person-centred care.
>
> So, what can health care leaders do to counteract this epidemic? IHI believes an important part of the solution is to focus on restoring joy to the health care workforce.'

While, at a first glance, this might seem implausible, a number of people are taking on this challenge, and the IHI offers some practical advice for leaders (see Figure 8.7). A practical example of how an organisation can improve joy at work is given in Figure 8.8.

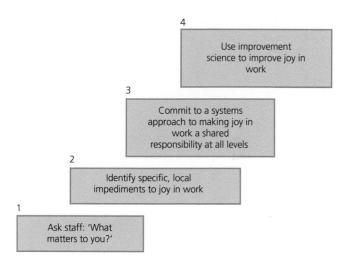

Figure 8.7 Four steps for leaders. Source: Adapted from Perlo *et al.* (2017).

What matters to you?	• Being able to take leave when I want to.
	• Feeling valued and supported by the organisation in my work.
	• Patient safety.
Identify specific local impediments	• Rotas initially had the lowest number of junior doctors at the busiest time of day (the evening shift).
	• Sick leave was relatively high for trainees at 4.3% – locums had to be contracted at short notice to fill gaps.
	• Night teams often came on duty to a back-log of work, which delayed assessments of patients.
Commit to a systems approach	• A rota was designed using a 'supply and demand framework', which reinforced the evening shift, reducing delays in patient assessment.
	• The rota was scrutinised and agreed with every level of doctor the changes affected.
	• Trainee engagement was valued, leading to a high level of support for the proposed changes when implemented.
	• The rota included increased capacity for annual leave.
Use improvement science	• These changes resulted in organisational benefits, including an 86.5% reduction in monthly expenditure on locums and improved seven-day staffing.
	• Sick leave fell from 4.2% to 0.3%.
	• Qualitative feedback from trainees was that they felt more supported during the evening and night shifts under the new system.
	• Senior clinicians reported a reduction in stress as clinical tasks were performed in a timely matter, simultaneously improving the patient experience.

Figure 8.8 A practical example of improving joy at work: redesigning junior doctor rotas (United Lincolnshire Hospitals NHS Trust, UK).

Conclusions

In recent years, the conversation has shifted from 'burnout' to 'moral injury' in order to better reflect the contribution of teams, organisations and the wider healthcare context to clinician burnout. In response to this, organisational kindness and compassionate leadership have become part of a national and international conversation and are inextricably linked to productivity and patient outcomes. In addition to basic 'housekeeping' responsibilities, focussing on Herzberg's hygiene factors and motivators, some have gone a step further, introducing the concept of 'joy at work'. It is clear that strategies to build satisfaction, motivation and even joy are beneficial to patients, profits and staff – but strategies that focus on individuals alone are not effective; a kind healthcare organisation has to focus on several levels and utilise all its available resources – key among these, *leadership* – to make organisational kindness a reality.

Further reading/resources

The Berwick Report (2013) A promise to learn – a commitment to act: improving the safety of patients in England. *National Advisory Group on the Safety of Patients in England*. Department of Health and Social Care. London.

Civility Saves Lives. Available at: www.civilitysaveslives.com (accessed June 2020).

Dean, W., Talbot, S. and Dean, A. (2019) Reframing clinician distress: moral injury not burnout. *Federal Practitioner*, **36** (9), 400–402.

Edwards, N. (2010) The triumph of hope over experience. Lessons from the history of reorganisation. *NHS Confederation*. Available at: www.nhsconfed.org/~/media/Confederation/Files/Publications/Documents/Triumph_of_hope180610.pdf (accessed June 2020).

Ferlie, E.B. and Shortell, S.M. (2001) Improving the quality of health care in the United Kingdom and the United States: a framework for change. *The Milbank Quarterly*, **79** (2), 281–315.

General Medical Council. (2019) Good Medical Practice. Updated April 2019. Available at: https://www.gmc-uk.org/ethical-guidance/ethical-guidance-for-doctors/good-medical-practice (accessed June 2020).

Herzberg, F. (2003) One more time: how do you motivate employees? *Harvard Business Review*, **81** (1), 87–96.

Maslach, C., Jackson, S.E. and Leiter, M.P. (1996–2016). *Maslach Burnout Inventory Manual*, 4th edition. Mind Garden Inc., Menlo Park, CA.

Perlo, J., Balik, B., Swensen, S. *et al.* (2017) *IHI Framework for Improving Joy in Work. IHI White Paper*. Institute for Healthcare Improvement, Cambridge, Massachusetts. Available at: http://www.ihi.org/resources/Pages/IHIWhitePapers/Framework-Improving-Joy-in-Work.aspx (accessed June 2020).

Porath, C.L. and Pearson, C. (2013) The price of incivility. *Harvard Business Review*, **91** (1–2), 114–121, 146.

Reimagining Better Medicine. Available at: https://fixmoralinjury.org (accessed June 2020).

Schein, E. (1985) *Organizational Culture and Leadership*. Jossey-Bass, San Francisco.

CHAPTER 9

Resilience in Practice

Carrie Krekoski and Victoria Wood

Office of the Vice President, Health, University of British Columbia, Canada

---

OVERVIEW

- Our ability to work effectively within today's team-based practice environments can be affected by our resilience and well-being.
- Effective teamwork contributes to our resilience and well-being, while ineffective relationships can have a negative impact.
- Trust, respect and effective communication are needed to ensure that teams and individual team members thrive.
- Interpersonal gaps can create conflict and reduce our resilience.
- Finding the most respectful interpretation is a strategy that can improve our interpersonal relationships.
- Psychological safety is about giving candid feedback, encouraging generative ideas, openly admitting mistakes and learning from each other.

Introduction

Healthcare professionals have always faced unique challenges and stressors, by virtue of the fact that they practice in a complex system (Braithwaite *et al.*, 2009). As with anyone, their ability to manage those stressors is impacted by their resilience and well-being. In today's healthcare setting, healthcare professionals practice in an environment where they face challenges that are too complex to be addressed by one profession alone, for example, the growth in the prevalence of chronic disease, cancer, mental health and substance use issues (Aggarwal and Hutchison, 2012). As such, healthcare professionals are increasingly expected to practice within team-based models of care, which can bring both benefits and challenges concerning provider resilience and well-being (Figure 9.1).

Effective teams can have a positive impact on provider resilience and well-being. However, when done ineffectively, working as part of a team can also have a negative impact on one's resilience and well-being. Collaboration with others requires effective interpersonal relationships that involve the exchange of information, coordination of processes, and shared decision-making, where there is an explicit underlying value of non-hierarchical collaboration. This may not always exist in practice.

Within today's team-based practice environments, trust, respect and effective communication are needed to ensure that teams and individual team members thrive. This chapter starts by discussing some of the ways in which low resilience can impact team interactions. We provide examples and case histories that span the continuum of practice, starting with the student experience. We highlight the fact that poor team functioning, which can impact patient care, is usually the result of ineffective communication that can stem from individuals who are languishing. We then introduce a communication strategy that promotes effective communication and psychological safety.

Individual resilience and practice

It is essential to start by recognising that healthcare professionals, as with everyone else, have a life outside their practice too. Lack of sleep, poor nutrition, interpersonal conflicts and trauma are just a few of the things in our everyday lives that can impact our resilience and well-being (Figure 9.2). We then bring this with us into practice, where the inherent stressors of healthcare can play a compounding role. This, in turn, may affect our relationships within the team and, subsequently, patient care.

What is 'team resilience'?

Resilience is described as an individual's ability to bounce back from negative emotional experiences or misfortune and to be able to demonstrate several positive psychological and behavioural characteristics when under duress (Luthans *et al.*, 2006; Gupta and Bonanno, 2010). At the individual level, resilience is characterised most often as adaptive responses within the individual. At the team level, resilience is associated with collective behaviours by team members and organisational processes that support collective behaviours resulting in positive adaptation (Pollock *et al.*, 2003; Bowers *et al.*, 2017). There is considerable literature that explores and measures individual resilience; however, research into the resilience of teams is just starting to emerge (Salas *et al.*, 2018).

ABC of Clinical Resilience, First Edition. Edited by Anna Frain, Sue Murphy, and John Frain.
© 2021 John Wiley & Sons Ltd. Published 2021 by John Wiley & Sons Ltd.

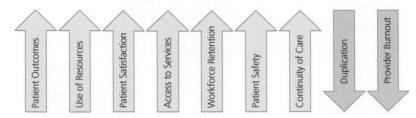

Figure 9.1 Why team-based care? Sources: Aggarwal and Huchinson (2012); Helfrich *et al.* (2014); Khan *et al.* (2008); Morgan *et al.* (2015).

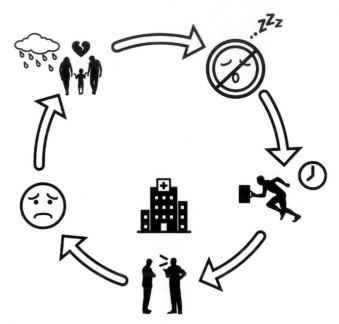

Figure 9.2 The cycle of diminishing resilience.

The impact on patient care

Patients dealing with complex issues often have multiple healthcare professionals who contribute to different aspects of their care (Box 9.1).

Processes and remuneration models often do not support collaboration, which can place the onus on individual healthcare professionals to communicate and collaborate with others involved in the care of their patients. When these efforts are perceived as a burden, it can impact a healthcare provider's willingness to communicate and collaborate, consequently impacting patient care.

Teams need to work together effectively to ensure they provide consistent messaging and recommendations, reduce duplication and coordinate care. When structures and processes in healthcare

---

> **Box 9.1 Team-based care.**
>
> 'The provision of comprehensive health services to individuals, families, and/or their communities by at least two health professionals who work collaboratively along with patients, family caregivers, and community service providers on shared goals within and across settings to achieve care that is safe, effective, patient-centered, timely, efficient, and equitable'.
>
> Source: Mitchell *et al.* (2012). ©2012, Project HOPE: The People-to-People Health Foundation, Inc.

> **Box 9.2 Case study – 'Who do I listen to?'**
>
> George, a 76-year-old man who just had knee replacement surgery, is eager to be discharged.
>
> His physical therapist, Samir, is covering patients for a colleague who is off sick. Claire, his occupational therapist, has a sick daughter at home and arrived late at work. Samir and Claire both arrive in George's room at the same time to discuss his discharge plan. George's daughter is there with him. Samir tells them that once George can walk 50 feet, which he is progressing towards nicely, he can be discharged. Claire interjects and suggests that she can get him home right away by fitting him for a wheelchair. George is confused and turns to his daughter in frustration, unclear on which recommendation to follow.

---

do not support collaboration, healthcare professionals may feel challenged to find the time and space, within already busy practices, to collaborate with other members of the team. This can have a cyclical effect on team resilience and well-being. Providers who feel burdened by the time it takes to communicate and collaborate with others may be less likely to do so (Box 9.2). This may then lead to ineffective patient care. When providers do not share consistent messaging with patients and families, this may reduce their trust in their healthcare team. As such, patients may be less likely to follow the advice of their healthcare providers, which can then impact the healthcare provider's perceptions about their own effectiveness and thereby lead to further reduced resilience and well-being.

Hierarchy and conflict

Healthcare structures and processes may also reflect historical hierarchies where the 'perceived status of individual team members can potentially disrupt team harmony with issues of authority, power and autonomy' (Hall and Weaver, 2001). It is possible that 'some healthcare professionals have more difficulty than others moving from a traditional hierarchy of professional roles and responsibilities to working with other disciplines in a more collaborative style' (Health Council of Canada, 2009). This can lead to conflict within teams and has the potential to impact the resilience and well-being of individual team members negatively. It is here that trust, respect and effective communication are essential, as unresolved conflict affects not only team functioning but also patient care (Box 9.3).

We need to work together to support team resilience and well-being. Within this context, effective communication can help foster

Box 9.3 **Case study – 'Who do you think I am?'**

Jamal is a new hygienist in Leila's dental practice. They have been working together for three weeks now, and Jamal is finding the way things are done to be very different from the last office he worked in. He loved working there, as he had an independent practice that allowed him to set his own hours. Leila likes a more collaborative approach, and Jamal often finds himself scheduled to work alongside Leila on complex cases. Every other Monday, Leila schedules a team meeting in the morning that Jamal needs to attend, even though Jamal only works afternoons and evenings. Today, Jamal is seeing a patient with Leila and is irritable because he had to miss his morning yoga class. When Leila asks him to order new gauze, Jamal snaps and curtly reminds her that that is not his job, before realising the patient is looking up at him in horror.

empathy and understanding amongst team members. One team member may need to contribute flexibility and understanding concerning the challenges associated with finding common time for team meetings. Other team members may need to be empathetic and supportive of other team members' schedules and the need for self-care.

The student experience

The impact of low resilience on our professional practice can start during training, where interprofessional education (IPE) is being integrated into health professional programs across the world as a mechanism to build the collaborative competencies that support team-based care (Thistlethwaite, 2012). This type of training often takes place in the practice setting and is an add-on to already full curricula. As such, students may enter these ses-

Box 9.4 **Case study – 'Not another interprofessional learning session!'**

Nadia is a third-year nursing student who has been busy studying all week for an upcoming exam that she is worried she will not pass. The exam is Friday, and she has been on placement all week, not getting time to study during the day. She has only had six hours of sleep cumulatively over the past two nights and has been living off vending machine food and coffee. Thursday afternoons are usually protected in her curriculum for group study time. However, this month, her program has scheduled interprofessional group learning sessions at her placement site during this time. At today's session, during which she has been placed in an interprofessional group of six students and assigned a complex ethical case to discuss, Nadia finds herself unwilling and unable to contribute to the case and expresses her frustration at the fact that this session is a complete waste of her time. In this moment, she feels like these interprofessional sessions will not contribute anything to her future practice. After the session, the other members of the group discuss how disrespectful nurses are, and that it is disgusting that they are not committed to collaborating with other professions.

sions with low resilience, resulting from the pressures of being in a demanding healthcare professional program (Box 9.4). However, IPE is an important mechanism for developing the effective communication needed to build resilient teams, as each health profession brings its own 'specialised vocabulary, similar approaches to problem solving, common interests and understanding of issues' (Hall and Weaver, 2001) that need to be understood and appreciated by others. Ineffective communication and interpersonal interactions within the context of such practice-based learning can have a detrimental effect on team cohesion in the long term.

Both health professional programs and students need to consider strategies that support student resilience and well-being. This is a stressful time that can have a profound impact on a student's well-being. The demands of health professional programs often result in poor eating and lack of sleep, which are integral to one's resilience and well-being (see Chapters 5 and 10).

Perception vs intention: bridging the interpersonal gap

Communication is foundational to conflict management, as well as individual and team resilience. The *Interpersonal Gap* model partially explains the potential for misunderstandings between team members (Figure 9.3). It refers to the degree of congruence between one person's intention and the effect produced in the other. If there is better fidelity between the effect and what is intended, the gap is bridged. The emotional impact of the interaction becomes considerable when the interpersonal gap is greater between what was intended and the receiver's interpretation. This model explains that each of us has intentions in every interaction with others; we encode our intentions into words and gestures; and the receiver decodes our words and actions to arrive at their interpretation. Their decoding determines the congruence of the message and the initial emotional impact the message has on them.

For example, while I may say, 'I am adjusting Mr. Smith's dosage today', intending to validate and endorse the change as positive, the receiver may interpret my message to mean that they made a mistake. The receiver may feel upset by this interpretation because she was planning on adjusting the dosage. The next time we interact, her perceptions of me are going to be filtered by her previous interpretation, and she may avoid me to circumvent a future insult. In this case, I did not clearly state my intention, and she did not say, 'Oh, what do you mean by that?' This type of interpersonal gap between healthcare providers can have a significant impact on team members and patient care.

We bring our personal filters that are influenced by our histories, assumptions, biases and preferences to every interaction. These are factors that filter our intentions and interpretations of messages received, and the opportunity for harmful interactions are everywhere. This is particularly salient in interprofessional teams because we use different languages (discipline-specific language) and have different approaches to patient care. We can close the interpersonal gap by checking in with each other about the words we use and our intentions before we jump to making some assumptions that undermine the interprofessional team.

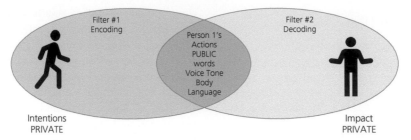

Figure 9.3 The interpersonal gap. Source: Based on Wallen (1967).

Most respectful interpretation

Most respectful interpretation is a strategy for bridging the interpersonal gap. It is one way in which teams can suspend judgement and build a supportive culture that recognises that people's behaviour may be the result of low resilience, rather than a negative intent (Russell *et al.*, 2007). This approach suggests that you consider only the best, the kindest, the most helpful interpretation of every communication and respond solely to that version (Box 9.5). The respectful interpretation we choose does not need to be accurate, but by reacting based on this interpretation, our actions change in a way that leads to more positive interactions.

Most respectful interpretation involves making one's thinking and reasoning more visible to others and inquiring into others' thinking and reasoning. It is a quality of listening and interaction that enables groups to function effectively. It assumes positive intent and frees us to focus on listening to one another. We fre-

---

Box 9.5 **Case study – The most respectful interpretation.**

Sunah is working with a team to care for a particular patient and needs information from Mary before she can meet with the patient. Unable to reach her, Sunah sends Mary an email. When Mary does not respond, Sunah leaves her several voice messages. She suddenly remembers that, the last time they worked together, she and Mary had some disagreements. Sunah, therefore, concludes that Mary is avoiding her communications. As the days roll by, Sunah convinces herself that Mary is trying to sabotage her. As she recalls, Mary never liked her. She decides then and there that, the next time Mary needs something from her for a patient, she will not give it to her!

Alternatively, by adopting the philosophy of most respectful interpretation, Sunah can improve her communication and relationship with Mary through reflection and by becoming more aware of her own thinking and reasoning.

Using this approach, Sunah starts by observing the situation as objectively as possible – Mary did not return her email. Sunah then thinks of as many possible reasons for the situation and Mary's behaviour – Mary is off sick; Mary did not get her email; Mary is ignoring her, etc. By suspending judgment and choosing the most respectful interpretation, Sunah is more likely to respond in a positive way. The next time Sunah sees Mary, she asks, 'Did you get my email? I know some of the computers around here have been acting up. I became concerned when I did not hear back from you'. In response, Mary apologises and lets Sunah know that she has been off work with a family emergency, forgot to put an out-of-office message on, and has not checked her email for over a week.

---

quently judge ourselves by our good intentions but may attach negative interpretations to others' actions. That dual standard may lead to unwarranted mistrust that can undermine progress and create unnecessary stress. By adopting this philosophy of *most respectful interpretation*, we assume the best of others.

Moral courage and psychological safety in teams

Approaches that diminish interpersonal gaps and support listening can enhance psychological safety in the work environment. Clark (2020) identifies four types of psychological safety:

1 *Inclusion safety*: inclusion to belong on the team and protecting everyone's safety
2 *Learner safety*: permission to learn and make mistakes without criticism
3 *Contributor safety*: permission to contribute to the team with autonomy
4 *Challenger safety*: permission to challenge the status quo (e.g., can speak up if they feel unsafe)

In healthcare, we most often focus on the latter three. These are about giving candid feedback, encouraging generative ideas, openly admitting mistakes and learning from each other. Psychological health and safety are increasingly important in healthcare teams, where patient safety cannot be compromised. Researchers have discovered that resilient teams report making more mistakes than other teams, mostly because they are more willing to discuss them (Edmondson *et al.*, 2016; Carmeli and Gittell, 2009; Sujan *et al.*, 2019). Psychological safety and trust can help team members in adapting rules and policies to meet the needs of specific situations; it facilitates the courage to speak up about trade-offs when static protocols and organisational targets jeopardise patient safety or health outcomes (Sujan *et al.*, 2019).

We tend to focus less on *inclusion safety*, which both contributes to and supports resilience and well-being, and is equally important.

Maintaining our resilience and well-being is difficult once we are in a state of distress. As such, there is value in team members feeling safe to provide peer support, to help us notice when we are challenged and to encourage us to pause. This involves asking 'What is needed right now?' in order to support each other to feel safer, calmer and more competent during times of distress. We can help each other by normalising distress as a common response to stressful times and develop strategies within the team to mitigate stressors (Box 9.6). Strategies such as Schwartz Rounds (see Chapter 7),

Box 9.6 **Case study – 'Are you okay?'**

Kalpen has worked in Zac's clinic for the past five years. The clinic team is very collegial and tries to take time to get to know each other on a personal level. They have a potluck lunch once a month, a barbeque in the summer with everyone's families and a holiday party each December. While Kalpen maintains a professional distance, not sharing much about his personal life, he attends these social functions and has a friendly working relationship with all the clinic staff. He has always been a conscientious employee who stays on top of his work and responds to issues quickly and professionally. However, Kalpen has lately been slow to respond to emails, is often late for work and seems to be paying less attention to his personal hygiene. While Zac wants to respect Kalpen's privacy, he is concerned about these changes in behaviour. He decides to take Kalpen for lunch, which he does often with clinic staff, to broach the subject. He asks, 'How are you doing? I have noticed some changes in your behaviour and am worried. I just want you to know that I am here. Just let me know what you need'. It turns out that Kalpen is a single father, and his daughter has been having some learning challenges. He feels relieved at being able to talk about it with Zac, and they decide to change Kalpen's schedule so he can pick his daughter up from school and be around for her in the afternoons.

Box 9.7 **Think about. . .**

- Reflect on a time when you had an interpersonal gap or team conflict that might have been a result of low resilience.
- List some of the factors that undermine individual and team resilience.
- Identify some strategies to support team resilience.

where people have the opportunity to share their vulnerability and engage in dialogue with others about the heart of their work, can create a safe environment that fosters resilience and well-being.

Conclusion

Together, healthcare professionals are part of a health and healing community and should develop strategies and processes to support each other to be resilient practitioners. Team-based practice models have been found to improve patient outcomes and satisfaction; improve access to services; ensure patient safety; improve continuity of care; improve workforce retention; reduce duplication; use healthcare resources more efficiently; and reduce provider burnout (Aggarwal and Hutchison, 2012; Helfrich *et al.*, 2014; Khan *et al.*, 2008; Morgan *et al.*, 2015). These outcomes and a team culture of trust, respect, open communication and psychological safety create an environment that fosters practitioner resilience and well-being. Communications theory such as the *interpersonal gap* and approaches such as the *most respectful interpretation* help us recognise that the intent of what we say does not always equal the intended effect on the listener. Likewise, our interpretation of the other person's behaviour in the most respectful way allows us to suspend judgement, remain open and recognise that people's behaviour may be the result of low resilience or a misunderstanding rather than a negative intent. This, in turn, builds a culture of psychological safety amongst members of a team, within which they can support each other in a way that maintains resilience and well-being. Individual resilience is facilitated by teams and organisational processes which value each member of the team and support effective communication, inclusion, learner, contributor and challenger safety (Box 9.7).

Further reading/ resources

Aggarwal, M. and Hutchison, B. (2012) *Toward a Primary Care Strategy for Canada*. Canadian Foundation for Healthcare Improvement, Ottawa, Canada.

Bowers, C., Kreutzer, C., Cannon-Bowers, J. and Lamb, J. (2017) Team resilience as a second-order emergent state: A theoretical model and research directions. *Frontiers in Psychology*, **8**, 1360. DOI: 10.3389/fpsyg.2017.01360. PMID: 28861013; PMCID: PMC5562719.

Braithwaite, J., Runciman, W.B. and Merry, A.F. (2009) Towards safer, better healthcare: Harnessing the natural properties of complex sociotechnical systems. *BMJ Quality & Safety*, **18** (1), 37–41. DOI: 10.1136/qshc.2007.023317. PMID: 19204130; PMCID: PMC2629006.

Carmeli, A. and Gittell, J.H. (2009) High-quality relationships, psychological safety, and learning from failures in work organizations. *Journal of Organizational Behavior*, **30** (6), 709–729.

Chinmaya, A. and Vargo, J.W. (2012) Improving Communication: The Ideas of John Wallen. *Canadian Journal of Counselling and Psychotherapy*, **13** (3). Retrieved from https://cjc-rcc.ucalgary.ca/article/view/60255

Clark, T.R. (2020) *The 4 Stages of Psychological Safety: Defining the Path to Inclusion and Innovation*. Berrett-Koehler Publishers, Oakland, California.

Edmondson, A.C., Higgins, M., Singer, S. and Weiner, J. (2016) Understanding psychological safety in health care and education organizations: A comparative perspective. *Research in Human Development*, **13** (1), 65–83. DOI: 10.1080/15427609.2016.1141280

Gupta, S. and Bonanno, G.A. (2010) Trait self-enhancement as a buffer against potentially traumatic events: A prospective study. *Psychological Trauma: Theory, Research, Practice, and Policy*, **2** (2), 83–92. https://doi.org/10.1037/a0018959

Hall, P. and Weaver, L. (2001) Interdisciplinary education and teamwork: A long and winding road. *Medical Education*, **35** (9), 867–875. DOI: 10.1046/j.1365-2923.2001.00919.x. PMID: 11555225.

Health Council of Canada (2009) *Teams in Action: Primary Health Care Teams for Canadians*. Health Council, Toronto.

Helfrich, C.D., Dolan, E.D., Simonetti, J. *et al.* (2014) Elements of team-based care in a patient-centered medical home are associated with lower burnout among VA primary care employees. *Journal of General Internal Medicine*, **29** (2), S659–S666. DOI: 10.1007/s11606-013-2702-z. PMID: 24715396; PMCID: PMC4070238.

Khan, S., McIntosh, C., Sanmartin, C. *et al.* (2008) *Primary health care teams and their impact on processes and outcomes of care*. Statistics of Canada: Health Research *Working Paper Series*. Ottawa. ISSN: 1915-5190; ISBN: 978-0-662-48998-6

Luthans, F., Vogelgesang, G.R. and Lester, P.B. (2006) Developing the psychological capital of resiliency. *Human Resource Development Review*, **5** (1), 25–44. DOI:10.1177/1534484305285335

Morgan, S., Pullon, S. and McKinlay, E. (2015) Observation of interprofessional collaborative practice in primary care teams: An integrative literature review. International Journal of Nursing Studies, **52** (7), 1217–1230. DOI: 10.1016/j.ijnurstu.2015.03.008. Epub 2015 Mar 19. PMID: 25862411.

Pollock, C., Paton, D., Smith, L. and Violanti, J. (2003) Team resilience, in *Promoting Capabilities to Manage Posttraumatic Stress: Perspectives on Resilience* (eds D. Paton, J.M. Violanti, L.M. Smith, pp. 74–88). Charles C Thomas Publisher.

Russell, C.K., Gregory, D.M., Care, W.D. and Hultin, D. (2007) Recognizing and avoiding intercultural miscommunication in distance education: a study of the experiences of Canadian faculty and aboriginal nursing students. *Journal of Professional Nursing*, **23** (6), 351–361.

Salas, E., Zajac, S. and Marlow, S.L. (2018) Transforming health care one team at a time: Ten observations and the trail ahead. *Group & Organization Management*, **43** (3), 357–381. DOI:10.1177/1059601118756554

Stress First Aid Self Care/Organizational Support Model. Available at: https://www.theschwartzcenter.org/media/Stress-First-Aid-Self-Care-Organizational-NCPTSD10.pdf

Sujan, M.A., Huang, H. and Biggerstaff, D. (2019) Trust and Psychological Safety as Facilitators of Resilient Health Care. *Working Across Boundaries: Resilient Health Care, Volume 5* (pp. 125–136). Boca Raton, Florida: CRC Press

TeamSTEPPS Canada™. Available at: https://www.patientsafetyinstitute.ca/en/education/TeamSTEPPS/Pages/default.aspx (accessed 11.01.2021).

Thistlethwaite, J. (2012) Interprofessional education: A review of context, learning and the research agenda. *Medical Education*, **46** (1), 58–70. DOI: 10.1111/j.1365-2923.2011.04143.x. PMID: 22150197.

Wallen, J.L. (1967) *The Interpersonal Gap*. Northwest Regional Educational Laboratory, Portland, OR.

Wynia, M.K., Von Kohorn, I. and Mitchell, P.H. (2012) Challenges at the intersection of team-based and patient-centered health care: Insights from an IOM working group. *JAMA*, **308** (13), 1327–1328. DOI:10.1001/jama.2012.12601

CHAPTER 10

Can We Really Teach Resilience, Intelligent Kindness and Compassion?

Sue Murphy and Betsabeh Parsa

Faculty of Medicine, Department of Physical Therapy, University of British Columbia, Vancouver Campus, Canada

---

OVERVIEW

- Resilience is increasingly considered a professional attribute which can be taught and learned during the formal curriculum.
- Enhancing resiliency is a complex process affected by the dynamic interactions among personal, interpersonal and environmental factors.
- A curriculum for teaching resilience must consider the dynamic interplay among factors on all three levels.
- Teaching self-care, reflection and mindfulness (through lectures, workshops or programmes) are the most common forms of resilience training.
- The development of strong human relationships (with clients, supervisors, mentors and peers) and providing social supports are key factors in resilience development.
- Contextual change is an important aspect of developing resilience.

Introduction

The development of resilience, along with empathy, have only recently become areas of interest in health professional training programs. With growing complexity, demanding workloads and chronic stress in the healthcare environment, higher levels of resilience, or the ability to cope with adversity and 'bounce back' from a stressful situation, is becoming increasingly necessary to avoid burnout. Resilience is an important factor in improving the quality of patient care and safety (Eley *et al.*, 2016), and it is also needed for the development and maintenance of elements of professionalism such as altruism, communication, empathy and compassion for clients. Resilience was originally considered an individual trait, largely developed by personal experience of life events and by parenting styles, and was therefore assumed to be something that students developed before entering health professional training. Only recently has resilience been considered as a process that can be learned, and attention paid to its development during the formal curriculum; a shift likely made due to the overwhelming number of studies globally demonstrating high levels of stress and burnout in both learners and practicing clinicians (e.g., Hariharan and Griffin, 2019).

The nurturing and development of resilience in training programs is challenging. Enhancing resiliency is a complex process affected by the dynamic interaction of various factors on several levels. The complex interactions among factors that influence resilience make it one of the most difficult concepts to teach. To create effective interventions and training programs to enhance resilience, multiple factors that influence how learners function in a stressful situation must be considered.

Dynamic interactions among factors on personal, interpersonal and environmental levels allow individuals to successfully cope with and bounce back from stressful situations, and to use these situations for personal growth and development.

Personal factors

Personal factors (or internal resources) are considered the most important factors in building resilience. These factors include the attributes and characteristics of individuals that help them cope with stressful situations and include personal traits (i.e., self-esteem, self-efficacy, self-regulation, mindfulness, optimism, creativity and adaptability), coping style (i.e., active coping style) and lifestyle (i.e., self-care, maintaining physical activity and work–life balance) (Box 10.1).

While it can be argued that some personal traits are more suited to the development of resilience than others (a person who is naturally creative, for example, may find it easier to develop resilience), many personal factors (such as self-esteem) can be further developed and taught as part of the curriculum. Mindfulness (which influences resiliency by reducing the level of stress and burnout, improving psychological well-being, increasing self-control and enhancing communication skills) is becoming increasingly common as part of entry-level health professional curricula, as well as part of continuing professional development (Fox *et al.*, 2018). Lifestyle is another area which is often modifiable.

Box 10.1 Personal factors.

Joe Smith is on the first day of his first clinical rotation. He has not been a strong student academically and has had to retake a couple of exams. He is very nervous and is worried that he does not have the requisite skills and may harm a patient, despite his instructor's reassurance that he is ready for his first rotation.

Joe is helping a patient from bed to chair on his first morning, and the patient unexpectedly faints, despite Joe having checked their blood pressure and taken all recommended safety precautions prior to the transfer. Joe is devastated, as he is sure it is his fault, and begins to feel he is not well suited to a career in healthcare.

In this situation, Joe already has low self-esteem due to his academic weakness; diminished optimism about his ability to be successful on the rotation; and likely a lack of creativity and adaptability in this situation due to his inexperience. The reaction of his supervisor to the incident will be very important in determining whether resilience is developed or diminished. Using tools such as reflection, reinforcement for what was done correctly and putting the incident in context (i.e., that this was unexpected and unpredictable) will help to build resilience and self-efficacy, whereas an accusatory attitude or a lack of exploration of Joe's perceptions and feeling about the incident will tend to diminish it.

Interpersonal factors

Interpersonal factors are also important for the development of resilience. This includes factors such as connectedness and supportive social networks. Connections with others inside and outside professional practice, and levels of both actual and perceived social support from peers, team members and supervisors, play a protective role and increase an individuals' ability to cope with adversity. Communication skills are important at the interpersonal level as the ability to engage with social supports requires effective communication skills. Abilities in developing and maintaining professional, peer and family support along with social connectedness, positive role modelling and mentorship can be key strategies in developing resilience at the interpersonal level.

The personal and interpersonal aspects of resilience are closely linked, since many personal factors are shaped by interpersonal interactions and experiences. High levels of social support have been positively associated with a more effective coping style, optimism, self-esteem and motivation. *Perceived* social support (i.e., knowing the help is available if needed) also strongly influences psychological well-being and resilience.

Contextual/environmental factors

Recently, there has been a greater focus on the interactions among the personal and the contextual or environmental factors in promoting resilience. As Tusaie and Dyer (2004) pointed out, 'resilience does not function uniformly and automatically, but waxes and wanes in response to contextual variables'. These environmental and contextual factors can include the culture of academia and the culture of the workplace, as well as the hidden curriculum which includes unwritten social and cultural values, rules, assumptions and expectations.

Figure 10.1 provides a visual presentation of how we see the dynamic interactions among the three levels of factors that influence resilience. The dotted lines between the concentric circles represent the dynamic interaction between influential factors. Factors on the environmental level are often omnipresent and overarching, influencing all other levels of factors. Personal factors are not developed in a vacuum, but are impacted and influenced by factors on both interpersonal and contextual levels. For example, when investigating medical errors, or adverse events, organisations which have a 'learning culture' and consider the systematic factors leading to the error (such as high workloads or inadequate training) will likely invoke higher levels of resilience in their employees than an organisation whose culture is blame and punishment.

Developing the curriculum

A curriculum for teaching resilience must take into account the personal-, interpersonal- and contextual-level factors and the dynamic interplay among them. Although, in practice, these factors and levels are inter-related, we present strategies for teaching and learning each factor as a separate section for ease of understanding.

Personal level

Internal resources or personal-level factors are some of the most important elements in developing resilience. Resilience workshops, small-group problem-solving and discussions, simulation-based interventions, narrative videos and self-directed modules are helpful tools for developing skills at this level. Curriculum for addressing personal-level factors should also include cognitive and psychological interventions focusing on mindfulness and relaxation, and on improving self-esteem, self-regulation, self-awareness, self-care and self-efficacy.

Mindfulness can be taught in a number of formats, including mindfulness programs (e.g., 8–10-week programs in mindfulness-based stress reduction), lectures and workshops. Taking care of personal needs such as nutrition and sleep can be modelled in the curricula by designing schedules and cognitive learning loads that allow students to practice setting a work–life balance. Promoting awareness on self-care and the importance of self-management can also be achieved by asking students to journal their daily activities, or by small-group discussions of how the students have brought joy to their lives in recent weeks (Box 10.2).

Self-regulation and self-awareness can be developed by enhancing reflection capacities through reflective writing workshops or encouraging peer group reflection. Enhancing self-efficacy (i.e., individuals' belief and confidence in their ability to act in a way that impacts a situation and generates a desired outcome) requires more self-directed learning approaches, achieved by giving students more choice and control over aspects of their learning. Frequent constructive feedback also assists learners in building confidence and developing their sense of self-efficacy. Box 10.3 describes some recommended interventions for enhancing resilience on the personal level.

Examples of interventions focusing on the personal level

Teaching resiliency through psychosocial skills and mindfulness-based interventions is one of the most common forms of resilience training (Fox *et al.*, 2018). The Stress Management and Resiliency

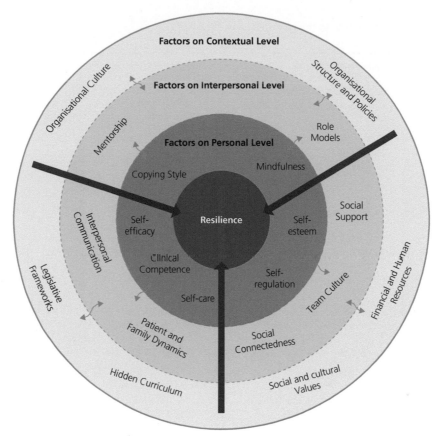

Figure 10.1 Visual presentation of interrelated factors influencing resilience.

Box 10.2 **Teaching self-care.**

Many health professional training programs now include theoretical elements related to the importance of self-care and work–life balance. However, the practical demands of these same programs often tell a different story, with a schedule of classes all day; 'extracurricular' tutorials and presentations during lunch breaks or in the evenings; and considerable homework expectations (including preparing for tests and exams). Modelling self-care by building breaks into the day where students are encouraged to exercise rather than participate in additional study, or by creating learning assignments such as asking students to journal their wellness activities (including diet, exercise and sleep routines) as part of a course, can all help students learn the art of self-care.

Training (SMART) program developed by Dr. Amit Sood in 2010 is one example of a resilience-enhancing intervention that has been utilised for enhancing resiliency in various populations (i.e., nurses, medical and nursing students, medicine faculty and breast cancer survivors) (Box 10.4). The SMART program was adapted from Attention and Interpretation Therapy (AIT), which was developed to reduce stress and increase resilience based on two aspects of human experience: attention and interpretation (Sood et al., 2011). The key component of the program is integration of mindfulness practices into everyday life, and principles of the program include attention training and the foundations of resilient thinking: gratitude, compassion, acceptance, meaning and forgiveness.

Interpersonal level

It has been suggested that meaningful contact with people acts as a catalyst for growth, and the development of strong human relationships with clients, supervisors, mentors and peers is an important factor in increasing resilience. Although it is acknowledged that there is a strong influence of social and interpersonal factors on resilience, how resilience is learned through social relationships is largely unclear. The ideal educational and clinical environment for developing resilience should foster the development of professional relationships, as well as social connections with peers and mentors. For example, peer mentoring, or the mentorship of junior students by senior students, appears to decrease students' distress and burnout (Fares et al., 2016) (Box 10.5).

Confident and supportive role models who demonstrate self-efficacy, control and individual responsibility are a key factor in developing resilience. Students' attitudes, beliefs and behaviour develop through observing and emulating the values and behaviours of role models in both academic and clinical contexts. Despite their important position in shaping students' resiliency, role models may be largely unaware of when or how they demonstrate resiliency, or how to encourage students to debrief and reflect in order to build resiliency (Box 10.6).

Providing counselling and academic accommodations (e.g., extension to coursework deadlines, additional time for writing exams or providing additional rest periods during clinical rotations) are important social support strategies for helping students navigate challenges and preventing burnout. It is worth noting, however, that providing too much support can put students at a

Box 10.3 **Recommended interventions based on the personal level of resilience.**

Theme	Underlying assumption	Suggested strategies
Mindfulness	Mindfulness increases self-monitoring and self-regulation, the factors associated with resilience	*Providing*: • Meditation workshops • Mindfulness and relaxation training
Self-care	The ability to care for self reduces stress and anxiety and increases resilience	*Encouraging students & professionals to*: • Set limits on work hours • Improve physical health and take care of personal needs such as sleep and nutrition • Find time for exercise and leisure activities
Reflection	Reflection fosters resilience through self-awareness, self-monitoring and self-regulation; the more professionals are aware of their emotions, strengths, weaknesses and vulnerabilities, the better they are positioned to become resilient	*Offering*: • Interactive reflective writing workshops • Creative writing workshops *Encouraging*: • Alternative forms of reflections such as peer group reflection sessions, artworks, online discussion boards, social networking sites and digital multimedia
Self-efficacy	One's confidence in her/his ability to solve problems is associated with resilience	• Considering the importance of feedback to build confidence • Using less didactic and more self-directed learning • Giving students some choice and control over aspects of their learning • Engaging and involving students with faculty in changing, designing and promoting programs
Problem-solving and coping mechanism	The use of approach-oriented coping strategies in problem-solving is related to mental health and resiliency	*Encourage following steps in problem-solving*: 1. Identify problems and define them 2. Investigate necessary resources 3. Develop strategies to solve the problems 4. Monitor the process 5. Evaluate the strategy after it is done
Psychosocial skills training	Internal resources, such as learned psychosocial skills, are necessary aspects of resiliency	Providing training related to: • Goal-setting skills • Stress-management • Constructively responding to criticism • Cognitive reframing • Self-compassion • Appreciation and gratitude

Box 10.4 **Example of intervention focusing on the personal level using the SMART program.**

Harry is a social work student in the emergency department. He is assessing an elderly patient who yells at him and 'wants to see a proper doctor, not some do-good student'. Harry is offended and hurt by the interaction and debriefs with his supervisor. Through reflection and discussion, Harry works through the steps of the 'SMART' program:
• *Gratitude*: Harry appreciates the learning experience as he will need to learn to deal with challenging behaviours and be able to set limits and boundaries.
• *Compassion*: Harry realises the patient is alone, scared and in pain.
• *Acceptance*: Harry accepts that these types of interactions may be 'part of the job', and that he will encounter many challenging individuals throughout his working life.
• *Meaning*: Harry reflects on the need to address not only the patient's pain and physical symptoms but to also provide reassurance and support as part of his care, and to build trust as part of the therapeutic relationship.
• *Forgiveness*: Although difficult, Harry is able to put the incident into context, and to not take the comments personally.

Box 10.5 **Examples of peer mentoring.**

Examples of peer mentoring in the clinical setting:
• Creating a 'community of practice'* for mentorship and support
• Buddy or mentoring programs
• Case rounds presented by team members
• Journal clubs
• Team huddles

Examples of peer mentoring in the educational setting:
• Small-group discussion
• Presentation of case studies
• Problem-based or case-based learning models
• Reflective exercises
• Interprofessional learning
• Debriefing with peers after clinical encounters

* Wenger (2011), defines *communities of practice* 'groups of people who share a concern or a passion for something they do and learn how to do it better as they interact regularly'.

disadvantage, as the complex and unpredictable environment of healthcare is usually filled with setbacks and struggles (Stoffel and Cain, 2018). To promote resilience, a delicate balance must be maintained between the level of stress and support (Box 10.7). Health professional educators need to proactively help students see stressors as potentially stimulating elements that are beneficial for learning, since an appropriate level of stress is linked to enhanced motivation and the development of skills in seeking support when needed (Box 10.8). Allowing students some experience of how to struggle, fail and recover, while increasing their communication skills and learning how to access help, is considered an effective approach in developing resilience.

Examples of interventions focusing on both personal and interpersonal levels

To our knowledge, there have not been many resilience training interventions that focus on both personal and interpersonal levels. The MaRIS model (Box 10.9) for developing resilience integrates four different levels into curriculum design (Chan *et al.*, 2020). The following section briefly describes the model; more information can be found in Chan *et al.* (2020).

Box 10.6 **Suggestions on developing resilience during clinical supervision.**

The following features are reported as factors contributing positively to resilience during clinical supervision:
1 *Normalisation*: Acknowledging the difficulty of the situation.
2 *Role modelling*: Talking about similar emotionally challenging experiences that the supervisor has had and the effective approaches that she/he took.
3 *Taking an exploratory approach*: Listening to learners and providing a space for them to develop their individual approach.
4 *Belief in the learner's capacity*: Providing implicit comments that demonstrate recognition of the learner's strengths.
5 *Assurance of backup*: Assuring learners that they are supported and not alone.
6 *Communicating the big picture*: Reminding students of the larger structure of their learning.

Source: Adapted from van den Engh and Veerapen (2020).

Box 10.7 **Stress and support: how to keep balance.**

A student is on the final rotation before graduation. The student has performed well throughout their training, but have always had a small caseload and patients with relatively simple problems. In the last rotation, the supervisor gives the student a larger caseload, as well as some challenging patients who have complex and non-traditional needs. The student initially finds this overwhelming and, in the first few days, the supervisor has to step in to ensure all the required care is provided. With the supervisor's support, however, the student learns better time management skills, and also what resources are available for new or challenging situations; they also experience how to ask for help in an effective way. The student is largely independent by the end of the rotation.

Box 10.8 **Recommended interventions based on interpersonal levels of resilience.**

Theme	Underlying assumption	Suggested strategies
Interpersonal and communication skills	Social and emotional connectedness and communicating effectively with the team and patients increase resilience	Providing workshops and training programs that focus on increasing communication and interpersonal skills
Role modelling	Role models are the keys to cultivating resilience	*Creating faculty development that:* • Helps academic and clinical faculty gain insights on resilience • Highlights their position as role models
Reflection	Since the influence of role models is not always positive, students need to have a high level of reflective competence that enables them to consider and reject unprofessional behaviours observed in role models	*Offering*: • Interactive reflective writing workshops • Creative writing workshops *Encouraging*: • Alternative forms of reflections such as peer group reflection sessions, artworks, online discussion boards, social networking sites, digital multimedia and school publications
Professional relationships and networks	Building positive, nurturing relationships and networks increase resilience	*Encouraging*: • Activities that reinforce a warm relationship in the educational and healthcare environment • Participation in professional community activities • Student-led support groups
Dialogue	There is a supportive benefit from sharing, discussing and critically reflecting upon common experiences, challenges and insights from adversity	Dedicating specific time for dialogue among all teams (students, faculty, health professionals, etc.) to share stories and resilient lessons learned from their experiences

Box 10.9 **The MaRIS model for developing medical students' human capabilities and personal resilience.**

MaRIS is a model developed to support medical students to enhance their human capabilities and personal resilience. It integrates *Mindfulness*, affective *Reflection*, *Impactive* experiences and a *Supportive* environment into medical curriculum design. Through this model, students engage in *mindfulness* practice and *affective reflection*, whilst being exposed to emotionally *impactive* (simulated) clinical experiences delivered in a *supportive* and safe environment.

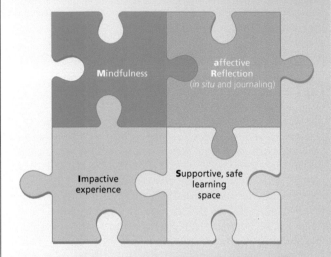

An example of this could be integrating mindfulness and guided reflection into supportive and safe debriefing sessions following exposure to clinical cases related to suicide or assisted dying.

Source: Based on Chan *et al*. (2020). © 2020, Taylor & Francis.

Contextual level

Although factors on the personal level play the most important role in promoting resilience, it is the appropriate culture and environment that promote and reinforce personal traits such as levels of self-care and help-seeking behaviour. The process of developing resilience, therefore, involves much more than what may be explicitly or implicitly learned during training workshops and intervention programs. Resilience develops through a process that internalises the moral, social and cultural values of a specific context; students internalise these norms within the educational process, and clinicians during their daily practice. For example, an educational or healthcare culture where seeking help is considered as a sign of weakness rather than an empowering act would be a deterrent to help-seeking behaviour (Box 10.10). Promoting resilience may therefore require contextual change; creating environments that are safe for failure, encourage help-seeking behaviour and have a culture of kindness and support can go a long way towards developing resilience in healthcare professionals (Box 10.11). In the educational setting, incorporating student feedback and perspectives into curricular development can, in addition to making the teaching more relevant, also empower students by developing self-esteem and self-efficacy, which builds resilience.

Box 10.10 **Contextual/ environmental factors.**

Asma Bakshi graduated a couple of months ago and is working at her first job in an outpatient wound care clinic. After her patient leaves, she realises she has given them the wrong supplies for the dressing changes at home; the dressings she supplied are cheaper but not as effective as the ones the patient should have had. She tells her supervisor that she will call the patient and ask them to come and collect the correct ones. Much to her surprise, the supervisor laughs and tells her not to worry about correcting the error, as 'the ones you gave her are fine and will save us some money'. She also advises Asma not to say anything about the error, as 'it doesn't really matter, and we don't want to look stupid'. Asma knows the correct dressings would be much more beneficial for the patient and feels that, not only is the quality of care being compromised, but she is being told that staff 'not looking stupid' and saving money are more important than optimal patient care. This is stressful for Asma as she feels she must hide her mistakes in future, and also leads to moral distress, in that she feels she cannot provide the best care for her patients. These factors can both lower resilience and predispose to burnout.

Examples of a model focusing on all personal, interpersonal and contextual levels

We are unaware of any resilience training interventions based on the dynamic interactions among all influential factors – although a proposed model, the Multi-System Model of Resilience, or MSMR (Box 10.12), examines the dynamic nature of the resilience process and considers three systems of influential factors (Liu *et al*., 2017). More than proposing recommendations about how to develop resilience, this model aims to address limitations in resilience research and capture the complexity of resilience. Box 10.12 briefly describes the model; more information can be found at Liu *et al*. (2017 and 2020).

Assessment of resilience

As attention to teaching and learning resilience is growing, the assessment of resilience development becomes important. The fact that resilience is a multi-dimensional, dynamic and complex construct makes it hard to measure. Assessing resilience requires a multi-dimensional and multi-system approach (Box 10.13). However, to date, the majority of proposed methods for measuring resilience have been focused on the personal level and psychological factors (Liu *et al*., 2017). The focus of measurement methods on personal factors without considering other relational and contextual variables creates a significant limitation to these measures. It is generally accepted that there is currently no 'gold standard' amongst measures of resilience, and that the complexity of resilience is not yet fully measured by existing methods (Windle *et al*., 2011).

In a methodological review of resilience measurement scales, Windle *et al*. (2011) identified 15 measures that propose to measure resilience. They, however, believed that all those measurement scales had some missing information regarding the

Box 10.11 **Recommended interventions based on contextual levels of resilience.**

Theme	Underlying assumption	Suggested strategies
Attention to the culture of the institution	Contextual factors play an underlying role in developing resiliency, and the faculty are key stakeholders for changing the context of the learning environment	*Providing faculty development*: To shift the culture so that self-care, cognitive and emotional awareness, and support-seeking behaviour are considered professional obligations
Reflection	Reflection helps students develop resilience by connecting their personal and interpersonal values to their experience in the context of the environment	*Offering*: • Interactive reflective writing workshops • Creative writing workshops • Opportunities for small-group debriefing or peer mentoring *Encouraging*: • Alternative forms of reflections such as peer group reflection sessions, artworks, online discussion boards, social networking sites, digital multimedia

Box 10.12 **Updated Multi-System Model of Resilience (MSMR).**

MSMR is a recent model proposed by Liu *et al.* (2017 and 2020) to capture the complexity of resilience. Highlighting the dynamic and multi-dimensional process of resilience, the updated MSMR includes "Internal Resilience" (sources of resilience within the individual),

"Coping & Pursuits" (coping-related skills that allow the individual to respond to challenges) and "External Resilience" (socio-ecological factors). The figure displays these three systems that act as the sources of resilience.

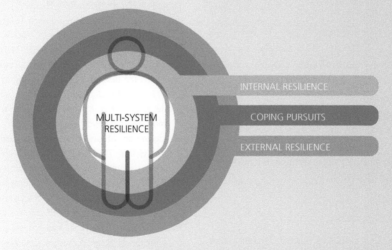

Source: Based on Liu *et al.* (2020). © 2020, Licensed under CC BY 4.0.

psychometric properties. Overall, they reported that the following scales received the highest rating:

- Connor–Davidson Resilience Scale (25 items)
- Resilience Scale for Adults (37 items)
- Brief Resilience Scale

Recently, two additional resilience measurement scales were developed to measure resilience at work and university:

- Resilience at Work (RAW) scale (Winwood *et al.*, 2013)
- Resilience at University (RAU) scale (Turner *et al.*, 2017)

Conclusion

Developing resilience is a complex process. The art and science of developing resiliency in clinicians and learners is in its infancy, and our understanding of how resiliency is learned is not fully developed. Providing best-practice recommendations on how to develop resilience among health professionals and health professional students is therefore challenging. A key message related to resilience training is that individuals are capable of learning resilience – but, since resilience is always contextual, a multifaceted approach must be used that includes focusing on individuals but also emphasises

> **Box 10.13 Four phases in assessing resilience interventions.**
>
> It is suggested that resilience training programs could be evaluated in the following four phases:
> - *Phase 1*: concept development and feasibility testing
> - *Phase 2*: trainings be tested in open-ended, uncontrolled studies
> - *Phase 3*: trainings be evaluated in randomised controlled trials (RCTs), which provide the most reliable evidence on the efficacy of interventions
> - *Phase 4*: larger field trials in real-world settings; after evidence for the efficacy of a multicomponent intervention has been established, studies should be conducted to identify effective training components
>
> Source: Adapted from Chmitorz *et al.* (2018).

> **Box 10.14 Key factors in the development of a 'resilience curriculum'.**
>
> - Taking a multifaceted approach incorporating the three levels of personal, interpersonal and contextual factors
> - Considering reflection as a key process in developing resilience
> - Including self-care, mindfulness and relaxation techniques, problem-solving and cognitive behavioural interventions
> - Providing social support, mentoring and peer mentoring
> - Paying attention to the effect of context

interpersonal relationships and institutional cultural change (Thompson *et al.*, 2016). Stand-alone methods that focus solely on one aspects of resilience (e.g., mindfulness) only capture a small section of a bigger picture. As suggested by Rogers (2016), reflection, mentoring, mindfulness and relaxation techniques, in combination with interventions targeting social and cultural levels, currently represent the best chance of success in fostering resilience in health professional students and clinicians (Box 10.14).

Further reading/ resources

Chan, K.D., Humphreys, L., Mey, A. *et al.* (2020) Beyond communication training: The MaRIS model for developing medical students' human capabilities and personal resilience. *Medical Teacher*, **42** (2), 187–195. DOI: 10.1080/0142159X.2019.1670340. Epub 2019 Oct 13. PMID: 31608726.

Chmitorz, A., Kunzler, A., Helmreich, I. *et al.* (2018) Intervention studies to foster resilience – a systematic review and proposal for a resilience framework in future intervention studies. *Clinical Psychology Review*, **59**, 78–100.

Eley, D.S., Leung, J., Hong, B.A. *et al.* (2016) Identifying the dominant personality profiles in medical students: Implications for their well-being and resilience. *PLoS One*, **11** (8), e0160028. DOI: 10.1371/journal.pone.0160028. PMID: 27494401; PMCID: PMC4975484.

Fares, J., Al Tabosh, H., Saadeddin, Z. *et al.* (2016) Stress, burnout and coping strategies in preclinical medical students. *North American Journal of Medical Sciences*, **8** (2), 75–81. DOI:10.4103/1947-2714.177299

Fox, S., Lydon, S., Byrne, D. *et al.* (2018) A systematic review of interventions to foster physician resilience. *Postgraduate Medical Journal*, **94** (1109), 162–170.

Hariharan, T.S. and Griffin, B. (2019) A review of the factors related to burnout at the early-career stage of medicine. *Medical Teacher*, **41**, 1380–1391.

Liu, J.J., Reed, M. and Girard, T.A. (2017) Advancing resilience: An integrative, multi-system model of resilience. *Personality and Individual Differences*, **111**, 111–118.

Liu, J. J., Reed, M., & Fung, K. P. (2020). Advancements to the Multi-System Model of Resilience: updates from empirical evidence. *Heliyon*, **6** (9), e04831.

Rogers, D. (2016) Which educational interventions improve healthcare professionals' resilience? *Medical Teacher*, **38** (12), 1236–1241.

Sood, A., Prasad, K., Schroeder, D. and Varkey, P. (2011) Stress management and resilience training among Department of Medicine faculty: a pilot randomized clinical trial. *Journal of General Internal Medicine*, **26** (8), 858–861.

Stoffel, J.M. and Cain, J. (2018) Review of grit and resilience literature within health professions education. *American Journal of Pharmaceutical Education*, **82** (2), 124–134.

Thompson, G., McBride, R.B., Hosford, C.C. and Halaas, G. (2016) Resilience among medical students: The role of coping style and social support. *Teaching and Learning in Medicine*, **28** (2), 174–182. DOI: 10.1080/10401334.2016.1146611. PMID: 27064719.

Turner, M., Holdsworth, S. and Scott-Young, C.M. (2017) Resilience at university: the development and testing of a new measure. *Higher Education Research & Development*, **36** (2), 386–400.

Tusaie, K. and Dyer, J. (2004) Resilience: a historical review of the construct. *Holistic Nursing Practice*, **18** (1): 3–10.

van den Engh, M. and Veerapen, K. (2020) Nurturing resilience in clinical supervision. *This Changed My Teaching (TCMT)*. Available at: http://thischangedmypractice.com/nurturing-resilience-in-clinical-supervision/

Wenger, E. (2011) Communities of Practice: A Brief Introduction. Available at: https://scholarsbank.uoregon.edu/xmlui/bitstream/handle/1794/11736/A%20brief%20introduction%20to%20CoP.pdf

Windle, G., Bennett, K.M. and Noyes, J. (2011) A methodological review of resilience measurement scales. *Health and Quality of Life Outcomes*, **9**, 8.

Winwood, P.C., Colon, R. and McEwen, K. (2013) A practical measure of workplace resilience: developing the resilience at work scale. *Journal of Occupational and Environmental Medicine*, **55** (10), 1205–1212. DOI: 10.1097/JOM.0b013e3182a2a60a. PMID: 24064782.

Recommended Books, Articles and Websites

For students and teachers

Ballatt, J., Campling, P. and Maloney, C. (2020) *Intelligent Kindness. Rehabilitating the Welfare State*. Cambridge University Press, Cambridge, UK.

Elton, C. (2018) *Also Human – The Inner Lives of Doctors*. Penguin Random House. **ISBN:** 9780099510796. London.

Harding, K. (2019) *The Rabbit Effect*. Atria Books.

Kalanithi, P. (2016) *When Breath Becomes Air*. Penguin Random House.

Markiewicz, L., West, M. and McKimm, J. (2017) Leading Groups and Teams", in *ABC of Clinical Leadership* (eds T. Swanwick and J. McKimm), Chapter 5. BMJ Books.

Sissay, L. (2019) *My Name Is Why. A Memoir*. Cannongate.

Walker, M. (2017) *Why We Sleep*. Penguin.

Academic

Aggarwal, M. and Hutchison, B. (2012) *Toward a Primary Care Strategy for Canada*. Canadian Foundation for Healthcare Improvement, Ottawa.

(The Berwick Report). (2013) A promise to learn – a commitment to act: improving the safety of patients in England. *National Advisory Group on the Safety of Patients in England*. Department of Health and Social Care, London.

Bohart, A.C. and Tallman, K. (1999) *How Clients Make Therapy Work: The Process of Active Self-Healing*. American Psychological Association, Washington DC. ISBN 10: 1557985715

Bourne, T., Vanderhaegen, J., Vranken, R. *et al.* (2016) Doctors' experiences and their perception of the most stressful aspects of complaints processes in the UK: an analysis of qualitative survey data. *BMJ Open*, **6** (7).

Bowers, C., Kreutzer, C., Cannon-Bowers, J. and Lamb, J. (2017) Team resilience as a second-order emergent state: a theoretical model and research directions. *Frontiers in Psychology*, **8**, 1360.

Braithwaite, J., Runciman, W.B. and Merry, A.F. (2009) Towards safer, better healthcare: harnessing the natural properties of complex sociotechnical systems. *BMJ Quality & Safety*, **18** (1), 37–41.

British Medical Association (BMA). (2020) *A Charter for Medical Schools to Prevent and Address Racial Harassment*. British Medical Association, London.

Burch, J.B., Alexander, M., Balte, P. *et al.* (2019) Shift work and heart rate variability coherence: Pilot study among nurses. *Association for Applied Psychophysiology and Biofeedback*, **44** (1), 21–30. DOI: 10.1007/s10484-018-9419-z. PMID: 30232570; PMCID: PMC6373270.

Carmeli, A. and Gittell, J.H. (2009) High-quality relationships, psychological safety and learning from failures in work organisations. *Journal of Organizational Behavior*, **30** (6), 709–729.

Casey, D. and Choong, K.A. (2016) Suicide whilst under GMC's fitness to practise investigation: Were those deaths preventable? *Journal of Forensic and Legal Medicine*, **37**, 22–27.

Chan, K.D., Humphreys, L., Mey, A. *et al.* (2020) Beyond communication training: The MaRIS model for developing medical students' human capabilities and personal resilience. *Medical Teacher*, **42** (2), 187–195.

Chancellor, J., Margolis, S., Jacobs Bao, K. and Lyubomirsky, S. (2018) Everyday prosociality in the workplace: The reinforcing benefits of giving, getting, and glimpsing. *Emotion*, **18** (4), 507–517.

Chemali, Z., Ezzeddine, F.L., Gelaye, B. *et al.* (2019) Burnout among healthcare providers in the complex environment of the Middle East: a systematic review. *BMC Public Health*, **19**, 1337.

Chmitorz, A., Kunzler, A., Helmreich, I. *et al.* (2018) Intervention studies to foster resilience – a systematic review and proposal for a resilience framework in future intervention studies. *Clinical Psychology Review*, **59**, 78–100.

Clark, T.R. (2020) *The 4 Stages of Psychological Safety: Defining the Path to Inclusion and Innovation*. Oakland, CA.

Colombo, B., Iannello, P. and Antonietti, A. (2010) Metacognitive knowledge of decision-making: an explorative study, in *Trends and Prospects in Metacognitive Research* (eds A. Efklides and P. Misailidi, pp. P445–472). Springer, New York, NY.

Coyle, D. (2009) *The Talent Code*. Arrow Books, London.

Croskerry, P. (2009) A universal model of diagnostic reasoning. *Academic Medicine*, **84** (8), 1022–1028.

Dean, W., Talbot, S. and Dean, A. (2019) Reframing clinician distress: moral injury not burnout. *Federal Practitioner*, **36** (9), 400–402.

Duma, N., Maingi, S., Tap, W. *et al.* (2019) Establishing a mutually respectful environment in the workplace: a toolbox for performance excellence. *American Society of Clinical Oncology Educational Book*, **39**, e219–226.

Durning, S.J., Costanzo, M., Artino, A.R. Jr, *et al.* (2013) Functional neuroimaging correlates of burnout among Internal Medicine Residents and Faculty Members. *Frontiers in Psychiatry*, **4**, 131.

Edmondson, A.C., Higgins, M., Singer, S. and Weiner, J. (2016) Understanding psychological safety in health care and educational organisations: A comparative perspective. *Research in Human Development*, **13** (1), 65–83.

Eley, D.S., Leung, J., Hong, B.A. *et al.* (2016, August) Identifying the dominant personality profiles in medical students: Implications for their well-being and resilience. *PLoS One*, **11** (8), e0160028. DOI: 10.1371/journal.pone.0160028. PMID: 27494401; PMCID: PMC4975484.

ABC of Clinical Resilience, First Edition. Edited by Anna Frain, Sue Murphy, and John Frain.
© 2021 John Wiley & Sons Ltd. Published 2021 by John Wiley & Sons Ltd.

Fox, S., Lydon, S., Byrne, D. *et al.* (2018) A systematic review of interventions to foster physician resilience. *Postgraduate Medical Journal*, **94** (1109), 162–170.

General Medical Council (GMC) (2019) *Caring for Doctors; Caring for Patients*. General Medical Council, London.

Ginsberg, J.P., Berry, M.E. and Powell, D.A. (2010) Cardiac coherence and PTSD in combat veterans. *Alternative Therapies in Health and Medicine*, **16** (4), 52–60.

Goodrich, J. (2011) *Schwartz Rounds - evaluation of the UK pilots*. The Kings Fund, London.

Gottlieb, M., Chung, A., Battaglioli, N. *et al.* (2020) Impostor syndrome among physicians and physicians in training: a scoping review. *Medical Education*, **54** (2), 116–124.

Hall, P. and Weaver, L. (2001) Interdisciplinary education and teamwork: A long and winding road. *Medical Education*, **35** (9), 867–875. DOI: 10.1046/j.1365-2923.2001.00919.x. PMID: 11555225.

Hariharan, T.K. and Griffin, B. (2019) A review of the factors related to burn-out at the early-career stage of medicine. *Medical Teacher*, **41**, 1380–1391.

Health Council of Canada (2020) *Teams in Action: Primary Health Care Teams for Canadians* (p. 14). Health Council, Toronto.

Hewitt, S. and Kennedy, U. (2020) *Wellness Compendium*. Royal College of Emergency Medicine, London.

Hofmann, P.B. (2018) Stress among healthcare professionals calls out for attention. *Journal of Healthcare Management*, **63** (5, September–October), 294–297.

Horsfall, S. (2014) *Doctors who Commit Suicide While Under GMC Fitness to Practice Investigation*. The General Medical Council, London.

Iannello, P., Mottini, A., Tirelli, S. *et al.* (2017) Ambiguity and uncertainty tolerance, need for cognition, and their association with stress. A study among Italian practicing physicians. *Medical Education Online*, **22**, 1.

Katz, D., Blasius, K., Isaak, R. *et al.* (2019) Exposure to incivility hinders performance in a simulated operative crisis. *BMJ Quality and Safety*, **28**, 750–757.

Kern, S., Oakes, T.R., Stone, C.K. *et al.* (2008) Glucose metabolic changes in the prefrontal cortex are associated with HPA axis response to a psychosocial stressor. *Psychoneuroendocrinology*, **33** (4), 517–529.

Khan, S., McIntosh, C., Sanmartin, C. *et al.* (2008) *Statistics of Canada: Health Research Working Paper Series*. Health Information and Research Division, Ottawa.

Kim, K. and Lee, Y.M. (2018) Understanding uncertainty in medicine: concepts and implications in medical education. *Korean Journal of Medical Education*, **30** (3): 181–188.

Kirby, J.N., Doty, J.R., Petrocchi, N. and Gilbert, P. (2017). The current and future role of heart rate variability for assessing and training compassion. *Frontiers in Public Health*, **5**, 40. https://doi.org/10.3389/fpubh.2017.00040

Land, R., Meyer, J.H.F. and Flanagan, M.T. (2016) *Threshold Concepts in Practice*. Sense Publishers, Rotterday, Taipei & Boston.

Lemaire, J.B., Wallace, J.E., Lewin, A.M. *et al.* (2011) The effect of a biofeedback-based stress management tool on physician stress: a randomized controlled clinical trial. *Open Medicine*, **5** (4), 154–163.

Liu, J.J., Reed, M. and Girard, T.A. (2017) Advancing resilience: An integrative, multi-system model of resilience. *Personality and Individual Differences*, **111**, 111–118.

Logan, T. and Malone, D.M. (2018) Nurses' perceptions of teamwork and workplace bullying. *Journal of Nurse Management*, **26** (4), 411–419.

Lown, B.A. (2016) A social neuroscience-informed model for teaching and practicing compassion in health care. *Medical Education*, **50** (3), 332–342.

Ludick, M. and Figley, C.R. (2017) Toward a mechanism for secondary trauma induction and reduction: reimagining a theory of secondary traumatic stress. *Traumatology*, **23** (1), 112.

Luthans, F., Vogelgesang, G.R. and Lester, P.B. (2006) Developing the Psychological Capital of Resiliency. *Human Resource Development Review*, **5** (1), 25–44.

Gupta, S. and Bonanno, G.A. (2010) Trait self-enhancement as a buffer against potentially traumatic events: a prospective study. *Psychological Trauma: Theory, Research, Practice, and Policy*, **2**, 83.

Mamede, S., van Gog, T., van den Berge, K. *et al.* (2010) Effect of availability bias and reflective reasoning on diagnostic accuracy among internal medicine residents. *JAMA*, **304** (11, September 15), 1198–1203.

Mann, K., Gordon, J. and MacLeod, A. (2009) Reflection and reflective practice in health professions education: a systematic review. *Advances in Health Science Education: Theory and Practice*, **14** (4), 595–621. PMID:18034364

Mathers, N. (2016) Compassion and the science of kindness: Harvard Davis Lecture 2015. *British Journal of General Practice*, **66** (648), e525–e527.

McBee, E., Ratcliffe, T., Picho, K. *et al.* (2017) Contextual factors and clinical reasoning: differences in diagnostic and therapeutic reasoning in board certified versus resident physicians. *BMC Medical Education*, **17** (1, November 15), 211.

McCraty, R. (2015) *Science of the Heart: Exploring the Role of the Heart in Human Performance, Volume* 2. HeartMath Institute, Boulder Creek, California.

Morgan, S., Pullon, S. and McKinlay, E. (2015) Observation of interprofessional collaborative practice in primary care teams: an integrative literature review. *International Journal of Nursing Studies*, **52** (7), 1217–1230.

Nijstad, B., De Dreu, C.K.W., Rietzschel, E.F. and Baas, M. (2010) The dual pathway to creativity model: creative ideation as a function of flexibility and persistence. *European Review of Social Psychology*, **21** (1), 34–77.

Norman, G.R. and Eva, K.W. (2010). Diagnostic errors and clinical reasoning. *Medical Education*, **44**, 94–100.

Olsen, E., Bjaalid, G. and Mikkelsen, A. (2017) Work climate and the mediating role of workplace bullying related to job performance, job satisfaction, and work ability: A study among hospital nurses. *Journal of Advanced Nursing*, **73** (11), 2709–2719.

Obholzer, A. and Roberts, V. (1994) *The Unconscious at Work*. Brunner-Routledge.

Pollock, C., Paton, D., Smith, L. and Violanti, J. (2003) Training for resilience, in *Promoting Capabilities to Manage Posttraumatic Stress: Perspectives on Resilience* (eds D. Paton, J.M. Violanti and L.M. Smith). Charles C. Thomas Publisher, Springfield, IL.

Porath, C. and Erez, A. (2011) How rudeness takes its toll. *British Psychological Society*, **24**, 508–511.

Porath, C.L. and Pearson, C. (2013) The price of incivility. *Harvard Business Review*, **91** (1–2), 114–121, 146.

Puddester, D., Flynn, L. and Cohen, J. (2019) *CanMEDS Physician Health Guide; A Practical Handbook for Physician Health and Well-being*. The Royal College of Physicians and Surgeons of Canada, Ottawa.

Raab, K. (2014) Mindfulness, self-compassion, and empathy among health care professionals: a review of the literature. *Journal of Health Care Chaplaincy*, **20** (3), 95–108.

Rendelmeir, D.A., Molin, J. and Tibshirani R.J. (1995) A randomised trial of compassionate care for the homeless in an emergency department. *Lancet*, **345**, 1131–1134.

Riley, K. and Gibbs, D. (2014) Revitalizing care program in UK Healthcare: does it add up? *Global Advances in Health and Medicine*, **3** (Suppl 1), BPA10.

Riskin, A., Erez, A., Foulk, T.A. *et al.* (2015) The impact of rudeness on medical team performance: a randomized trial. *Pediatrics*, **136** (3), 487–495.

Rogers, D. (2016) Which educational interventions improve healthcare professionals' resilience? *Medical Teacher*, **38** (12), 1236–1241.

Russell, C.K, Gregory, D.M., Dean, W. and Hultin, D. (2007) Recognising and avoiding intercultural miscommunication in distance education: A study of the experiences of Canadian faculty and aboriginal nursing students. *Journal of Professional Nursing*, **23** (6), 351–361.

Sacco, T.L. and Copel, L.C. (2018) Compassion satisfaction: a concept analysis in nursing. *Nursing Forum*, **53** (1), 76–83. https://doi.org/10.1111/nuf.12213

Salas, E., Zajac, S. and Marlow, S.L. (2018) Transforming health care one team at a time: Ten observations and the trail ahead. *Group & Organization Management*, **43** (3), 357–381. DOI:10.1177/1059601118756554

Schein, E. (1985) *Organizational Culture and Leadership*. Jossey-Bass, San Francisco.

Schön, D.A. (1983) *The Reflective Practitioner: How Professionals Think in Action*. Basic Books, New York.

Shirom, A., Toker, S., Alaky, Y. *et al.* (2011) Work-based predictions of mortality: a 20 year follow up of healthy employees. *Health Psychology*, **30** (3), 268–275.

Sinclair, S., (1997) *Making Doctors: An institutional apprenticeship*. Berg, Oxford.

Smith, J., Stewart, M., Foggin, S. *et al.* (2020) Schwartz Centre Rounds in second-year medical students using clinical educator-facilitator group work session: not just 'a facilitated moan"! *BMC Medical Education*, **20**, 271.

Smith, J.G., Morin, K.H. and Lake, E.T. (2018) Association of the nurse work environment with nurse incivility in hospitals. *Journal of Nurse Management*, **26** (2), 219–226.

Sood, A., Prasad, K., Schroeder, D. and Varkey, P. (2011) Stress management and resilience training among Department of Medicine faculty: a pilot randomized clinical trial. *Journal of General Internal Medicine*, **26** (8), 858–861.

Stenfors, C.U., Hanson, L.M., Theorell, T. and Osika, W.S. (2016) Executive cognitive functioning and cardiovascular autonomic regulation in a population-based sample of working adults. *Frontiers in Psychology*, **7** (October 5), 1536.

Stoffel, J.M. and Cain, J. (2018) Review of grit and resilience literature within health professions education. *American Journal of Pharmaceutical Education*, **82** (2), 124–134.

Sujan, M.A, Huang, H. and Biggerstaff, D. (2019) *Working Across Boundaries: Resilient Health Care*, Volume 5 (pp. 125–136).

Thistlethwaite, J. (2012) Interprofessional education: a review of context, learning and the research agenda. *Medical Education*, **46** (1), 58–70. DOI: 10.1111/j.1365-2923.2011.04143.x. PMID: 22150197.

Thompson, G., McBride, R.B., Hosford, C.C. and Halaas, G. (2016) Resilience among medical students: the role of coping style and social support. *Teaching and Learning in Medicine*, **28**, 174–182.

Thomas, C. and Quilter-Pinner, H. (2020) *Care Fit for Carers. Ensuring the Safety and Welfare of NHS and Social Care Workers During and After Covid-19*. Institute for Policy Research.

Tod, D., Hardy, J. and Oliver, E. (2011) Effects of self-talk: a systematic review. *Journal of Sport and Exercise Psychology*, **33** (5), 666–687.

Turner, M., Holdsworth, S. and Scott-Young, C.M. (2017) Resilience at university: The development and testing of a new measure. *Higher Education Research & Development*, **36**(2), 386–400.

Tusaie, K. and Dyer, J. (2004) Resilience: a historical review of the construct. *Holistic Nursing Practice*, **18** (1), 3–10.

van den Berge, K. and Mamede, S. (2013) Cognitive diagnostic error in medicine. *European Journal of Internal Medicine*, **24**, 525–529.

Wagaman, M.A., Geiger, J.M., Shockley, C. and Segal, E.A. (2015) The role of empathy in burnout, compassion satisfaction, and secondary traumatic stress among social workers. *Social Work*, **60** (3), 201–209.

Wayne, S., Dellmore, D., Serna, L. *et al.* (2011) The association between intolerance of ambiguity and decline in medical students' attitudes toward the underserved. *Academic Medicine*, **86**(7), 877–882.

Weinman, J., Ebrecht, M., Scott, S., *et al.* (2008) Enhanced wound healing after emotional disclosure intervention. *BJ Health Psychology*, **13**, 95–102.

Whitehead, B., Owen, P., Henshaw, L. *et al.* (2016) Supporting newly qualified nurse transition: a case study in a UK hospital. *Nurse Education Today*, **36**, 58–63.

Windle, G., Bennett, K.M. and Noyes, J. (2011) A methodological review of resilience measurement scales. *Health and Quality of Life Outcomes*, **9**, 8.

Winwood, P., Colon, R. and McEwa, E. (2013) A practical measure of workplace resilience: Developing the resilience at work scale. *Journal of Occupational and Environmental Medicine*, **35** (10), 1205–1212.

Wu, A.W. (2000) The doctor who makes the mistake needs help too. *BMJ*, **320**, 726.

Websites (all accessed November 2020)

Civility Saves Lives. Available at: www.civilitysaveslives.com.

GP-S. Available at: https://www.gp-s.org/.

For a (downloadable) audio demonstration of a validated self-regulation technique from the HeartMath Institute see: https://www.heartmath.org/resources/heartmath-tools/quick-coherence-technique-for-adults/ (accessed 17/01/2021).

Reimagining Better Medicine. Available at: https://fixmoralinjury.org (accessed June 2020).

Stress First Aid Self Care / Organizational Support Model. Available at: https://www.theschwartzcenter.org/media/Stress-First-Aid-Self-Care-Organizational-NCPTSD10.pdf

TeamSTEPPS Canada™. Available at: https://www.patientsafetyinstitute.ca/en/education/TeamSTEPPS/Pages/default.aspx

To learn more about the research behind heart coherence and its role in stress and emotional wellbeing see: https://www.heartmath.org/resources/videos/scientific-foundation-of-the-heartmath-system/

UK Resource for Schwartz Rounds. A group reflective practice forum which provides opportunities for staff from all disciplines to reflect on the emotional aspects of their work. Available at: https://www.pointofcarefoundation.org.uk/our-work/schwartz-rounds/

West, M. (2017) *Collaborative and Compassionate Leadership*. Available at: *https://www.kingsfund.org.uk/audio-video/michael-west-collaborative-compassionate-leadership* (accessed 12.08.2020).

Index